Massage Therapy Review

Passing the NCETMB and NCETM

Laura Abbott, MS, LMT, NCTMB
Premier Performance, Inc., Atlanta, Georgia

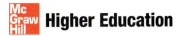 **Higher Education**

Boston   Burr Ridge, IL   Dubuque, IA   New York   San Francisco   St. Louis
Bangkok   Bogotá   Caracas   Kuala Lumpur   Lisbon   London   Madrid   Mexico City
Milan   Montreal   New Delhi   Santiago   Seoul   Singapore   Sydney   Taipei   Toronto

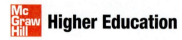

McGraw Hill **Higher Education**

MASSAGE THERAPY REVIEW: PASSING THE NCETMB AND NCETM

Published by McGraw-Hill, a business unit of The McGraw-Hill Companies, Inc., 1221 Avenue of the Americas, New York, NY 10020. Copyright © 2008 by The McGraw-Hill Companies, Inc. All rights reserved. No part of this publication may be reproduced or distributed in any form or by any means, or stored in a database or retrieval system, without the prior written consent of The McGraw-Hill Companies, Inc., including, but not limited to, in any network or other electronic storage or transmission, or broadcast for distance learning.

Some ancillaries, including electronic and print components, may not be available to customers outside the United States.

 This book is printed on recycled, acid-free paper containing 10% postconsumer waste.

4 5 6 7 8 9 0 QWD/QWD 0 9

ISBN 978-0-07-352073-5
MHID 0-07-352073-X

Publisher: *David T. Culverwell*
Developmental Editor: *Connie Kuhl*
Senior Marketing Manager: *Nancy Bradshaw*
Senior Project Manager: *Sheila M. Frank*
Senior Production Supervisor: *Kara Kudronowicz*
Designer: *Rick D. Noel*
Cover/Interior Designer: *John Rokusek*
Lead Photo Research Coordinator: *Carrie K. Burger*
Compositor: *Electronic Publishing Services Inc., NYC*
Typeface: *10/12 Giovanni Book*
Printer: *Quebecor World Dubuque, IA*

Photos not credited on page provided by author, Laura A. Abbott

Library of Congress Cataloging-in-Publication Data

Abbott, Laura A.
    Massage therapy review : passing the NCETMB and NCETM / Laura A. Abbott. – 1st ed.
      p. cm.
    Includes index.
    ISBN 0-07-352073-X—ISBN 978-0-07-352073-5 (alk. paper)
      1. Massage therapy–Examinations, questions, etc.   2. Masseurs–Certification–United States–Study guides.   I. Title.

RM721.A23 2008
615.8'22076—dc22   2006046974

www.mhhe.com

Dedication

Thank you to my wonderful husband, Justin, for his patience in waiting for me to finish this project before getting his massage; to my family, friends, and co-workers for dealing with my stress levels; to my students who teach me as much as I hope I teach them; and to my models (Justin, Ursula, Craig, Justin G., and Michael).

About the Author

Laura Abbott is an NCTMB licensed massage therapist who graduated from the Academy of Somatic Healing Arts in Atlanta, October 2000. She earned her undergraduate degree in Exercise Science in 1987 and her master's degree in Sports Medicine in 1988 from Georgia State University. She interned at Emory University Cardiac Rehabilitation and at Georgia Institute of Technology Athletic Department. Laura worked with Federal Occupational Health training and educated Federal Law Enforcement officers and traveled around the country presenting continuing education programs for many years. She has been quoted in *Ladies Home Journal* magazine (Nov. 2000) and was a featured speaker for the *Speaking of Women's Health Expo* for two consecutive years. Laura also has presented at the National American College of Sports Medicine Conference and currently teaches in the kinesiology and health department at Georgia State University, and in the massage therapy department at Georgia Medical Institute (Corinthian Colleges, Inc). She has owned and operated Premier Performance, Inc., in Atlanta since 1991 which specializes in exercise and massage rehabilitative therapies and continuing education programs. To learn more about Premier Performance, Inc visit the website at www.premier-performance.com.

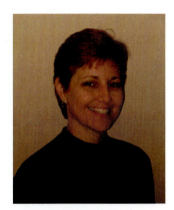

Laura Abbott

Brief Table of Contents

Table of Contents

Preface

Many years ago when I was fresh out of graduate school, I attended a national conference for fitness professionals. This conference was attended by thousands of people, mostly PhDs, so you can imagine how I felt surrounded by brilliant professors and research specialists in the field. While the presentations and research were wonderful, they never really answered my question: How can I incorporate findings from your lab into work with my clients?

Soon after, I was sent a survey about the conference. I expressed how wonderful it was, but I felt that I didn't really have information that I could take and apply to my workplace. To my surprise, I was asked to present the next year. The following year I presented on how to incorporate exercises for people with arthritis into the workplace, and how to translate the exercises into their daily activities—basically how to make their exercise more functional. The room seated only 100 people, and to my surprise about 300 people filled the room. When I returned to my hotel, it dawned on me—people don't want just the facts, they want to know how and why.

Fast forward several years to my completion of massage school. I finished (just like you) and it was now time for me to take my national exam. Although I found many useful study guides, I found one thing lacking: explanations to the questions. I didn't just want to know what I missed, I wanted to know why I missed it. So why not write a book to help people understand this information?

This book offers you a unique and valuable study tool. In June 2005, the organization of the NCBTMB test changed, and this is the first book to recognize that change. Before, NCBTMB only offered one test which included Eastern Modalities. When the organization realized that many schools did not offer courses in Eastern Modalities, they decided to offer two different tests, one with a focus on Eastern Modalities (NCETMB) and one without (NCETM). Also, emphasis was taken away from areas that, although important, were not a focus of a massage therapist. In addition, areas that are a huge focus for therapists, such as muscles and their structure, were increased. The organization of the book follows that of the new NCETM and NCETMB exams.

The six parts of this book correspond to the six parts of the exam which are
(1) general knowledge of body systems
(2) detailed knowledge of physiology, anatomy, and kinesiology
(3) therapeutic massage assessment
(4) therapeutic massage application
(5) pathology and
(6) professional standards, ethics, business and legal practices. The percentages at the beginning of each chapter correspond to the percentage weight of each section on the exam. There is a separate Eastern Modalities chapter (Chapter 7) because only the NCETMB exam covers this area.

In addition, the number of questions at the end of each chapter corresponds to the percentage weight of each section. Although these are not direct questions from the exam, as that would be a copyright infringement, but it gives you an idea of how questions might be asked. The format of the test assists you with the timing of the test. Remember, you have 140 questions and three hours to take it.

I now have several certifications under my belt and have investigated many workbooks, not only in massage, but in other areas of health. None of the study guides I found included all the areas I have provided for you in this book. Many books offered test questions and answers only, others only had the workbook. This book provides you with the study guide, questions, answers, and explanations. It doesn't help us to only know we missed the question, we need to know why the correct answer is what it is, and this book does that for you. This book also incorporates the needs of different types of learners. Having taught in the classroom for many years, I realize that part of my job includes accommodating and incorporating different learning styles. For those visual and kinesethic learners, this book has a fabulous selection of high quality artwork, photos, and drawings; something that you can't get from a book full of questions and answers. For those who are visual, this book has detailed text, charts and tables for your use. Mnemonic devises are also throughout various sections that offer another way to retain the information.

Each chapter ends with a selection of questions to test your knowledge. Not all of the questions are pulled directly from the study guide. Granted, there are many different types of massage schools and programs, but you will all have covered the material at some point in your education.

This book is designed to teach you how to prepare for the exam, provide focus and information on the areas of competency, and illustrate a thinking process so you can handle just about any question that comes your way. This book offers one-stop shopping for your national exam preparation. Memorizing only takes you so far in life, but knowledge knows no limits.

I hope that this book will benefit you and your career.

Laura Abbott, MS, NCTMB
Premier Performance, Inc
2897 N. Druid Hills Rd.
Suite 115
Atlanta, GA 30329
404-406-2873
www.premier-performance.com

To the Instructor

The national exam has six areas of competency on each of the two exams (NCETMB and NCETM). Both exams have parallel areas; Chapter 7 is designed to cover Eastern Modalities, which is found only on the NCTMB exam. The uniqueness of this book is that it not only reviews each area thoroughly, but it also tests the students' knowledge with end of the chapter questions and answers. Another unique factor is that each question comes with an explanation for yet another method of studying. The CD-ROM also adds over 900 questions, answers, and rationales for a more enhanced learning experience. The seven areas of competency are as follows:

Chapter 1 General Knowledge of Body Systems provides a thorough review of each of 11 body systems. This provides the basis for future chapters in this workbook and ensures a basic understanding of the human body.

Chapter 2 Detailed Knowledge of Anatomy, Physiology, and Kinesiology goes further into depth of the workings of the body, movement terminology, muscle contractions, and biomechanics. A list of muscle origins/insertions/actions is also included. Nutrition is introduced in this section.

Chapter 3 Pathology provides a more in-depth coverage of medical terminology, disease pathology and its affect and involvement with massage therapy.

Indications and contraindications are covered in the section as well as the healing process, and psychological stress, abuse, and approaches by other health care professionals. Pharmacology (prescription, recreational drugs, and herbs) is also covered in this section.

Chapter 4 Therapeutic Massage and Bodywork Assessment reviews endangerment sites, ergonomic factors, and the effects of gravity on the body.

Chapter 5 Therapeutic Massage Applications reviews the physiological, emotional, and psychological effects of massage. Methods and techniques of massage are also covered (draping, stress management techniques, and other holistic techniques) as well as massage techniques and strokes. Also covered are standard precautions, CPR, and basic first aid and safety.

Chapter 6 Professional Standards, Ethics, Business and Legal Practices reviews the NCBTMB Code of Ethics and other professional considerations when operating your practice.

Chapter 7 Eastern Modalities is only on the National Certification for Therapeutic Massage and Bodyworkers exam (NCTMB). It covers meridians, chakras, pathologies, and their relationship to Eastern Modalities, the physiology of meridians and channels, and basic Eastern Modality assessments.

Each chapter ends with questions, answers, and rationales for the section covered. Mnemonic devices, practical relationships, memory helpers, and At-A-Glance features are also helpful in students' comprehension of the material.

The comprehensive CD-ROM provides even more questions, answers, and rationales. The workbook and CD-ROM can be used for classroom or independent self-study.

To the Student

You've taken on the successful challenge of working to become a massage therapist and/or body worker; now it is time to focus on the national exam. It is important to know and understand how the body works from a physiological and anatomical sense, as well as how to run or manage a business, and of course, to perform massage. It seems overwhelming, but you know you can do it.

Remember, the national exam is actually two different exams. You get to choose which one you would like to take. The National Certification Examination for Therapeutic Massage and Bodywork (NCETMB) covers the basics of massage and also Eastern Modalities (Chapter 7 in this book). The National Certification Examination for Therapeutic

Massage (NCETM) covers the basics of massage only. Each chapter corresponds to an area of competence with a percentage weight on the national exam. At the beginning of each chapter you'll find a list of the details for each area of each exam according to the National Certification Board for Therapeutic Massage website www.ncbtmb.com.

With so many study guides out there to assist you, we are glad you have chosen this one. In investigating other study guides, we combined the format in order to best suit you. Included in this packet is a workbook that reviews each section of the national exam.

- Words that are **bolded** and/or underlined are words of importance. One should focus on these words, definitions, etc., in order to assist in the basic understanding of the area of discussion.
- Also in the workbook are "At-A-Glance" tables to help summarize important points. "Test-Taking Tips" and "Strategies to Success" will help you focus. "Memory Helpers" offer easy mnemonic means to memorize key points.
- At the end of each chapter you'll find review questions. Remember, understanding and application will help you build and retain your knowledge, and will also help you the day of the test!
- In order to help you further, the rationales for each question can be found at the end of the review questions. This will help you not only identify what you missed but help you understand why. Our goal is not only to succeed in passing the exam, but to succeed in your practice as well.
- This manual is designed to be used with the CD-ROM as a study guide and offers over 900 *more* questions, answers, and rationales to further your knowledge and understanding.

Study Tips

- Give yourself plenty of time to study. Cramming for any test is not beneficial. Make a time commitment each day to study. Put it on your calendar and schedule this time just like you would schedule a client.
- Know yourself and your study habits. What time of day are you the most productive? How long can you concentrate before you need a break? Where do you study best?
- Get a study partner. Maybe a former classmate is also studying for the exam. This can help you stay committed to your scheduled study times while providing another set of eyes, ears, and mind to digest the information.

Test Taking Tips

- Answer the question being asked—don't read too much into the question.
- Read the whole question before you answer.
- Studies show that going back and changing your answers is risky. Usually the answer is changed because you thought too much about the question!
- Relax!
- Get a good night's sleep the night before the test.
- Give yourself plenty of time to get to the testing center.
- Do not cram the morning/day of the test—you either know it by now or not. It will make you panic more if you try last minute cramming
- If you know and understand how the body works, you can figure out the answer. This is where memorizing is not as beneficial as being able to apply your knowledge.
- And did we say relax?!

Now you can begin the investment in your future as a massage therapist and/or body worker. We know you can succeed!

Walkthrough

To help the students prepare for NCETMB/NCETM exams each chapter opens with a list of the basic competencies and the percentage number of questions that will be asked on the test.

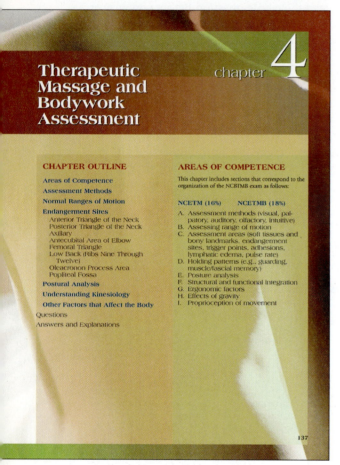

Therapeutic Massage and Bodywork Assessment — chapter 4

CHAPTER OUTLINE

Areas of Competence
Assessment Methods
Normal Ranges of Motion
Endangerment Sites
  Anterior Triangle of the Neck
  Posterior Triangle of the Neck
  Axillary
  Antecubital Area of Elbow
  Femoral Triangle
  Low Back (Ribs Nine Through Twelve)
  Oleacronon Process Area
  Popliteal Fossa
Postural Analysis
Understanding Kinesiology
Other Factors that Affect the Body
Questions
Answers and Explanations

AREAS OF COMPETENCE

This chapter includes sections that correspond to the organization of the NCBTMB exam as follows:

NCETM (16%)   NCETMB (18%)

A. Assessment methods (visual, palpatory, auditory, olfactory, intuitive)
B. Assessing range of motion
C. Assessment areas (soft tissues and bony landmarks, endangerment sites, trigger points, adhesions, lymphatic edema, pulse rate)
D. Holding patterns (e.g., guarding, muscle/fascial memory)
E. Posture analysis
F. Structural and functional integration
G. Ergonomic factors
H. Effects of gravity
I. Proprioception of movement

137

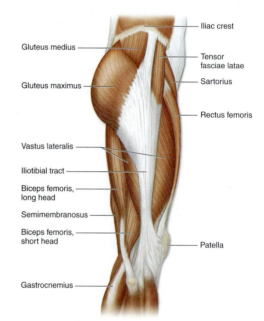

Dynamic illustrations lend a realistic view to enhance learning.

TABLE 2-10			
At a Glance: Muscles That Move the Thigh and Leg			
Muscle	Origin	Insertion	Action
Psoas major	Transverse processes and vertebral bodies of T12–L5	Lesser trochanter	Unilaterally: laterally rotates the hip Bilaterally: flexes the hip and the vertebral column
Iliacus	Iliac fossa and anterior inferior iliac spine	Lesser trochanter	Flexes and laterally roates the hip Flexes hip; extends hip
Gluteus maximus	Posterior sacum, posterior coccyx, and posterior iliac crest	Glutal tuberosity (25%) and iliotibial band (75%)	Extends, laterally rotates, and abducts the hip
Gluteus medius	Superior gluteal line	Greater trochanter	Abducts and medially rotates the hip Flexes hip; extends hip
Gluteus minimus	Inferior gluteal line	Greater trochanter	Abducts and medially rotates the hip, and flexes hip
Tensor fasciae latae	Anterior iliac crest and anterior superior iliac spine	Iliotibial band	Abducts, flexes, and medially rotates the hip

At-a-Glance tables help to summarize important information.

This book is well written with illustrations, tables, etc. to really help the students with studying.

Susan Bovo—Penn Commercial

Study Skills at the beginning of each chapter offer the students helpful tips for productive learning.

Test-Taking Skills at the end of every chapter provide students with practical tips to utilize for success.

Memory Helper boxes aid the students in recalling important concepts.

Questions

Therapeutic Massage Assessments
NCETM (16%) NCETMB (18%)

1. When massaging a child
   A. use towels as a top drape only.
   B. obtain written consent from both parents and child.
   C. have a parent supervise the massage session.
   D. ask the parent or guardian to wait outside the massage room.

2. A client with lordosis may experience a reduction in low back discomfort if a pillow is placed
   A. under the abdomen in the prone position.
   B. under the chest in the prone position.
   C. under the pelvis in the prone position.
   D. None of the above are correct.

3. In choosing the right kind of table, which of the following is not important?
   A. color
   B. comfort
   C. ergonomics
   D. ease of adjustment

4. Avoid massaging a new scar, especially after surgery, for
   A. seventy-two hours.
   B. one to two weeks.
   C. six to eight weeks.
   D. six months.

Answers and Explanations

NCETM (26%) NCETMB (26%)

1. **B** Remember, rubber bands are elastic and temporarily lengthen before going back to their original length. Plastic elongation is more permanent, like the plastic bottle that will maintain its shape. Therefore, elastic elongation is temporary and more for pre-event or pre-exercise with the goal of preparing you for exertional movement. Plastic elongation stretch is for post-exercise to help improve, in a more permanent way, flexibility.

2. **A** Think of your pelvis as a basin of water. Tilt the basin downward in the front, and the water spills out in front. If the pelvis does the same movement, this is an anterior pelvic tilt. In this case, the anterior superior iliac spine is tilted down or lower in front than the posterior iliac spine in back. This is commonly seen in people whose pants are higher in the back on the waist and low in front on the waist.

3. **D** The origin is the medial clavicle and the manubrium of the sternum. The insertion, which is the question, is the mastoid process.

4. **B** The posterior scalenes attaches to rib 2; the sternocleidomastoid attaches to the clavicle and the sternum, not to the ribs.

Review questions at the end of every chapter reinforce massage therapy competencies.

Answers and Explanations to each question ensure the students' understanding.

I have not seen a review book that was as well organized or with as many review questions and answers with explanations.

Michelle Burns—Advanced Holistic Healing Arts

Acknowledgments

I would like to thank Tony Hodge for helping me be in the right place at the right time; Kim Wyatt and George Stamathis for their intellect and insightfullness; Connie Kuhl and the rest of the McGraw-Hill staff who helped with this book—your dedication, detail, and conscientious efforts have been above and beyond. And a special thanks to all the reviewers who took the time to share their knowledge and expertise in each area of this book.

Reviewer

Denise M. Abrams, P.T., M.A.
Broome Community College
Binghamton, NY

Jodi Anderson
National American University
Roseville, MN

Mary Berger, BA, CMT
Kirtland Community College
Roscommon, MI

Paul V. Berry, Jr.
Lincoln Technical Schools
Norcorss, GA

Monique P. Blake
Keiser Career College
Miami Lakes, FL

Bernice Bicknase, Program Chair–Therapeutic Massage
Ivy Tech Community College of Indiana
Fort Wayne, IN

Raymond J. Bishop, Jr., Ph.D.
Rising Spirit Institute of Natural Health
Atlanta, GA

Paul Bolton, D.C.
National Holistic Institute
Emeryville, CA

Susan L. Bova, NCBTMB, Certified Master Medical Massage Therapist
Penn Commercial, Inc.
Washington, PA

Gregory J. Brink, LMT
University of Pittsburgh
Titusville, PA

Michelle Burns, BSRN, LMT, MTI
Advanced Holistic Healing Arts
Austin, TX

Karl "KC" Chambers, NCTMB/NMT, owner
Tenstrings A Healing Touch
Stone Mountain, GA

Virginia S. Cowen, Ph.D., L.M.T.
Queensborough Community College
Bayside, NY

Sheryl D. Daniel, BA, CMT, NMT, BMT, HNC, Reiki Master
Bear Mountain Massage Therapy and Holistic Health
    Institute
Greeley, CO

Mark L. Dennis, III, LMT, NCBTMB
Southern Massage Institute
Collierville, TN

Jennifer M. DiBlasio, AST, ACMT
Career Training Academy, Inc.
New Kensington, PA

Dana J. Douglas, NCTMB
Mt. Nittany Institute of Natural Health
State College, PA

Margaret F. Dutcher, RN, RMT
Virginia College
Jackson, MS

India Ferguson
Miller–Motte Technical College
Wilmington, NC

Ilyse T. Flattau, PT, MA
NYIT, Dept. of Physical Therapy
Old Westbury, NY

Lora Freeman
The Chicago College of Healing Arts
Chicago, IL

Jocelyn Granger
Ann Arbor Institute of Massage Therapy
Ann Arbor, MI

Kirsten Grimm
Vincennes University
Vincennes, IN

Carol Hainline, LMT, CNMT
Rising Spirit Institute of Natural Health
Atlanta, GA

Dave Henthorn, LMT, CAPT
Texas Massage Institute
Dallas, TX

Gregory Howie, BS, LMT, NCBTMTS
Birmingham School of Massage
Birmingham, AL

Robert J. Ianacone
Sonoma College
San Francisco, CA

Lisa Jakober, Corporate Director of Education
National Massage Therapy Institute
Philadelphia, PA

Jennifer Joseph
Colorado Institute of Massage Therapy
Colorado Springs, Co

Susan Kalchman, MT
American Institute of Massage Therapy
Santa Ana, CA

Judith Kennedy-Silcock
Magic Valley Academy of Massage
Twin Falls, ID

Mary E. Larsen, CAHI, CMT, RMA
Academy of Professional Careers
Nampa, ID

Julianne Lepp
Rising Spirit Institute of Health
Atlanta, GA

Joel Lindau
Cambridge College
Aurora, CO

Catherine A. Mastroianni, DC, CCSP
Ashmead College
Seattle, WA

Londyn Beck McGuigan
The Cittone Institute
Philadelphia, PA

Leigh A. Milne, RMT, RYT, PFT
Maui School of Therapeutic Massage
Makawao, HI

Jay M. Nelson, LMT, LMP (Member ABMP, NCBTMB)
Concorde Career Institute
Portland, OR

Cynthia Pavel, MPA, MT, CMT(NCBTMB), Dept Coordinator
School of Health Professions–Davenport University
Granger, IN

Carissa Pohlen
Minnesota West Community & Technical College
Pipestone, MN

Susan Pomfret, MA, LMT, Massage Therapy Program Coordinator
Central Arizona College
Apache Junction, AZ

Traci E. Quinton-Jones, NCMT
Georgia Career Institute
Conyers, GA

Dee Dee Roberts, CMT, CR
Boulder College of Massage Therapy
Boulder, CO

Holly Roche, BS, LMT
McIntosh College
Dover, NH

Charlene Herbert Russell, Massage Therapy Education Consultant
Blue Cliff/MTEC
Ocean Springs, MS

Dorothy J. Sala, LMT, CIMI
Teamwork, LLC.
Salem, CT

Suann Schuster, MA/L.C.M.T.
Great Lakes Institute of Technology
Erie, PA

David Lee Sessoms Jr. M.E.d., CMA
Miller–Motte Technical College
Wilmington, NC

Cheryl L. Siniakin, Ph.D., LMTI, NCTMB
Community College of Allegheny County
Pittsburgh, PA

Tina A. Sorrell, Director
American Institute of Allied Health
Lewisville, TX

Angela Staylor, Program Director
Virginia School of Technology
Richmond, VA

Sara J. Wallace
Miller–Motte Technical College
Wilmington, NC

Roxanna Woods, LMT
Health Works Institute
Bozeman, MT

Timothy P. Zembek, NCTMB
United Education Institute
Huntington Park, CA

Kevin C. Zorda, LMT
Branford Hall Career Institute
Windsor, CT

General Knowledge of Body Systems

chapter 1

CHAPTER OUTLINE

AREAS OF COMPETENCE

This chapter includes sections that correspond to the organization of the NCBTMB exam as follows:

NCTM (14%)

A. Anatomy
B. Physiology
C. Pathology*

- Integumentary (skin)
- Skeletal
- Muscular
- Nervous
- Endocrine
- Cardiovascular
- Lymphatic
- Urinary
- Respiratory
- Gastrointestinal
- Reproductive

NCBTMB (16%)

Content is the same as above with the following additions:

- Craniosacral
- Energetics
- Meridian

These fall under the Eastern Modality section and can be found in Chapter 7.

---

*Pathology will be covered in Chapter 3.

Strategies to Success

Study Skills

Organize and manage!

Organize your notes after class. Doing so will not only help you review material but will also make it easier to understand your notes when you go back to them to study for an exam. Organizing your notes right away will also give you plenty of time to ask your instructor to clarify something you didn't understand.

Anatomy and Physiology

Anatomy is the study of the parts of the body and its systems. Physiology is the study of how these parts and systems work. Understanding the parts helps us to understand the functions. Understanding the functions allows us to understand disease processes. So, let's begin by reviewing the major body systems and their functions.

Levels of Organization

The body, and all living things, have certain levels of organization. See Figure 1-1. Beginning at the cellular level, we can categorize these levels as follows:

Cells: Cells are the basic unit of all organisms. To be considered "living," an organism must breathe, ingest, excrete waste, generate energy, maintain itself, grow,

and reproduce. Cells do all of these. In fact, a cell is the smallest unit of life that can replicate itself. Cells consist of the cytoplasm, the cell membrane, and the nucleus.

Tissues: Tissues are a group of similar cells that perform similar functions. Four main categories of tissue are epithelial, connective, neural, and muscle.

Organ: An organ is a group of tissues that perform a similar specialized function. Such organs include the stomach, heart, lungs, liver, and gallbladder.

Organ system: An organ system is a group of organs that acts together to perform a specialized body function. The main organ systems are the circulatory, respiratory, digestive, integumentary, endocrine, nervous, skeletal, muscular, lymphatic, urinary, and reproductive systems.

Organism: This is an individual living thing.

Review of Major Body Systems

Massage therapists and body workers know and understand that what happens at the cellular level affects what happens to the organ system and vice versa. Let's take a look at the basic components and functions of the organ systems.

Integumentary: This system consists of the skin, hair, nails, and glands. The integumentary system provides support and protection. The skin is the largest organ in the body and makes up seven percent of body weight.

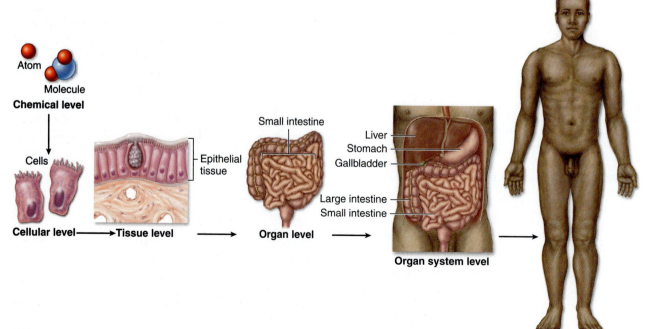

Figure 1-1 The human body is organized by levels, progressing from the cell to the organism.

Skeletal: This system provides support, protection, movement, generation of blood cells, and storage of minerals. The body contains 206 bones. The axial skeleton consists of the skull, vertebral column, pelvis, and rib cage. The appendicular skeleton consists of the upper and lower extremities.

Muscular: Connective tissue in this system creates muscle that helps to provide movement and body heat.

Nervous: This system includes organs such as the brain, spinal cord, and nerves that help the body to communicate and allow for memory and learning.

Sensory: This system includes the specialized organs (ears, nose, eyes, and tongue) which make it possible for us to hear, see, smell, and taste.

Circulatory: The circulatory system allows the body to receive nourishment via the blood as well as filter out waste and includes the heart and blood vessels.

Lymph: The lymph system helps the body with immunity, drains fluids from tissues, and filters waste via the lymph. This system includes the spleen, thymus, lymph nodes, and tonsils.

Respiratory: This system allows for the exchange of gases from the air into the body and bloodstream through the lungs, air passages, and alveoli sacs.

Gastrointestinal:
This system helps us to receive nutrients by taking in and digesting food which includes the stomach and intestines, as well as other organs.

Endocrine: The endocrine system secretes hormones that help to regulate homeostasis and body regulation. It includes such organs as the pancreas, pituitary, thyroid, adrenals, and gonads.

Urinary: The urinary system includes the kidneys, ureters, bladder, and urethra that work together to remove waste and excess water from the body.

Reproductive: This system allows for reproduction and includes the female uterus, ovaries, and vagina and the male testes, scrotum, and penis.

Energy Terminology

Metabolism: All of the chemical and physical processes that take place inside the body resulting in growth, production of energy, elimination of wastes, and other body functions are referred to as *metabolism*.

TABLE 1-1

At a Glance: Energy Terminology

Metabolic Aspects	Definition
Catabolism	The breakdown of substances into simple compounds that liberates energy for use in work and heat production
Anabolism	The conversion of simple compounds into more complex substances needed by the body
Homeostasis	When the body is in balance

The fundamental metabolic processes are catabolism and anabolism. See Table 1-1.

Catabolism: *Catabolism* is the destructive phase of metabolism. However, it can also be part of a normal process, such as normal bone growth and bone breakdown. Catabolism occurs when the body is stressed for long periods of time. Various systems are overworked and cannot keep up. The body begins to break down. For example, if the digestive system does not work well, we may get constipated. The thyroid may be overstressed, so it stops secreting hormones. Cortisol, a stress hormone, keeps secreting and the body begins to fall apart.

Anabolism: If and when the body begins the process of healing itself, it begins the constructive phase of metabolism called *anabolism*. As the body begins to heal, systems of the body begin to build back up and function again. However, anabolism can be negative as well. For example, a bone that continues to lay down more bone may cause a heel spur.

Homeostasis: When the body is in a process of equilibrium, as a result of the constant feedback and regulation, this is called *homeostasis*.

The Integumentary System

FUNCTION: Protection, temperature regulation, sensory reception, and cutaneous absorption (oxygen, carbon dioxide, sunlight).

Skin: There are three layers of skin: *epidermis*, *dermis*, and *subcutaneous*.

Epidermis: The most superficial layer of skin; this is what we physically touch when we massage. Two substances are found in the epidermis: *keratin* and *melanin*.

Keratin: Keratin is a protein found in the stratum corneum layer that makes the epidermis tough and impenetrable.

Melanin: Melanin is the dark pigment in the skin and hair that is produced by melanocytes. This is what protects us from the ultraviolet rays of the sun. It also explains why fair-skinned people are more likely to burn than those with darker skin.

Dermis: The dermis is the layer below the epidermis, composed of connective tissues, blood vessels, glands, muscle tissue, nerve endings, and hair follicles.

Subcutaneous: The subcutaneous layer is the deepest layer of the skin, composed mostly of connective tissues (mainly adipose or fat) and blood vessels.

Hair: The hair consists of a shaft, root, and bulb. Hair such as the eyelashes and nose hair offers limited protection, as well as sensory stimuli (such as in the ear).

Fingernails and toenails: These are the hardened layer of the stratum corneum. Nails are made of hard keratin. The lunula is the half moon located at the base of the nail. This is where nail growth takes place. Under the skin surface of our fingers and toes are the Meissner's corpuscles, which allow us to sense touch.

Mechanoreceptors are at the ends of neurons. They respond to mechanical pressure. The four main types are pacinian corpuscles, Meissner's corpuscles, Merkel's disc, and the tympanic membrane. Pacinian corpuscles are also known as Lemellated corpuscles, and are large receptors that detect deep pressure and vibration. They are found deep in the dermal layer of the skin, and the subcutaneous tissue of the palms of the hands and soles of the feet, the breast, and external genitalia. They are also found in the synovial membraned joints and in the walls of some organs.

Glands of the Integumentary System

There are three main types of glands within the integumentary system: *sebaceous* glands, *sudoriferous* glands, and *ceruminous* glands.

Sebaceous glands: Located along the hair shaft, these glands secrete sebum and help keep the stratum corneum supple and waterproof.

Sudoriferous glands: These are sweat glands that help to eliminate waste and help cool the body by removing heat through evaporation. (Sweat is ninety-nine percent water and one percent electrolytes and urea.) There are two main types of sudoriferous glands: eccrine and apocrine.

- **Eccrine glands**: Eccrine glands are the most numerous type of sweat glands, found primarily on the back, forehead, hands, and feet.
- **Apocrine glands**: These are the larger sweat glands in the axillary and pubic regions. These become active in puberty.

Ceruminous glands: Glands that secrete ear wax (cerumen).

The Skeletal System

FUNCTIONS: Storage of minerals, production of blood cells, protection, movement, and support. Three types of bone cells make up and maintain our skeletal system. See Table 1-2. There are five shapes of bones (*long, short, sesmoid, irregular,* and *flat*) and two types of bone tissue (*cancellous* and *compact*).

TABLE 1-2

At a Glance: Types of Bone Cells

Bone Cell	Description
Osteocytes	Individual bone cells
Osteoblasts	Cells that build up or repair bone tissue
Osteoclasts	Cells that break down bone tissue which helps release stored minerals

Bone Shapes

Flat bone: A flat bone consists of an outer covering of periosteum, a thin shell of compact bone, and an extensive inner core of cancellous bone. These bones, for example the ribs and skull, are generally for protection.

Long bone: Each long bone has a shaft called the *diaphysis*, which is composed of compact bone. Long bones also have two expanded ends called the *epiphyses* and a central canal (the medullary canal) within the diaphysis. Generally, one of the epiphyses is more rounded than the other and is called the head. Each epiphysis consists of a thin outer shell of compact bone and an extensive inner core of cancellous bone. These are generally found in the appendicular skeletal system and include bones such as the femur, radius, ulna, and humerus. See Figure 1-2.

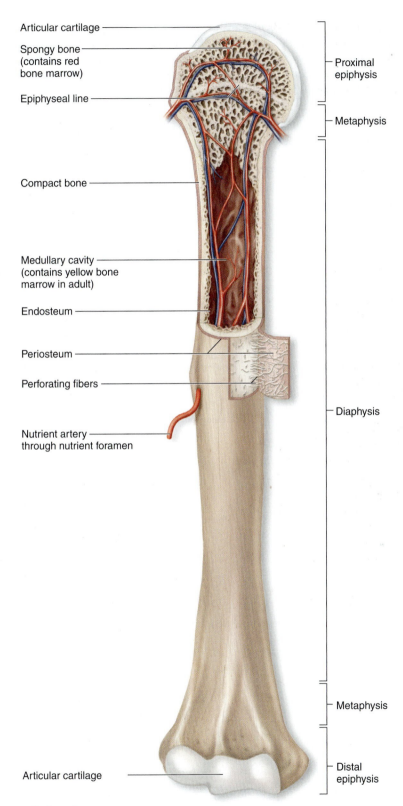

Articular cartilage

Spongy bone
(contains red
bone marrow)

Epiphyseal line

Compact bone

Medullary cavity
(contains yellow bone
marrow in adult)

Endosteum

Periosteum

Perforating fibers

Nutrient artery
through nutrient foramen

Articular cartilage

Proximal
epiphysis

Metaphysis

Diaphysis

Metaphysis

Distal
epiphysis

Figure 1-2 Major parts of a long bone.

Short: A short bone consists of an outer covering of periosteum, a thin shell of compact bone, and an extensive inner core of cancellous bone. Short bones are also generally found in the appendicular skeletal system and include such bones as the carpals and tarsals (Figures 1-3 and 1-4).

Irregular: These bones have the same basic construction as the flat and short bones except that they are highly irregular in shape. They are generally found in the axial skeletal system and include such bones as the vertebrae and pelvis.

Sesmoid: Sesmoid bones are typically tiny (like sesame seeds) and are found embedded in fibrous connective tissue in and around the joints. They are generally used for leverage, such as the patella and the sesmoid bone found at the base of the first metatarsal.

Bone Structure

Diaphysis: The diaphysis is the shaft of the long bone, composed mainly of compact bone.

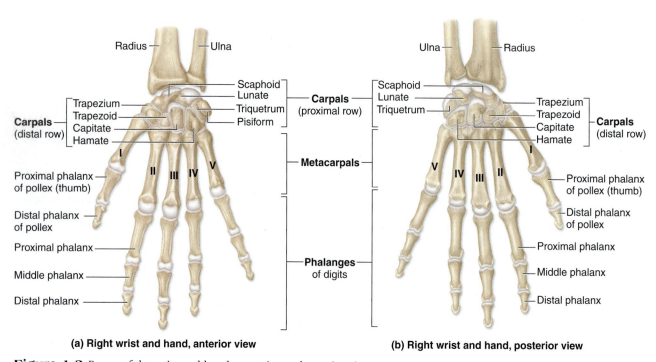

(a) Right wrist and hand, anterior view   **(b) Right wrist and hand, posterior view**

Figure 1-3 Bones of the wrist and hand, posterior and anterior views.

Memory Helper

The Carpal Bones
To remember the order of the carpals
starting with the proximal row
Sally Left The Party To Take Cathy Home

Epiphyses: This is found at either end of long bones. It is mainly composed of cancellous bone. This is also where you'll find the epiphyseal plates (or growth plates).

Periosteum: This is the layer of tissue that covers the bone surface. It is very rich in blood vessels and nerves. A broken bone is painful because it damages the nerves in the periosteum.

Medullary cavity: This cavity is in the diaphysis of long bones. In adults, it contains yellow bone marrow and is often called the marrow cavity.

Compact bone: Compact bone is the dense and heavy outer layer of the bone. The only openings in compact bone are tiny canals for blood vessels and microscopic cavities that contain osteocytes.

Cancellous bone: This is the spongy center of the bone found in the epiphyses of long bones which helps lighten the bone and absorb shock.

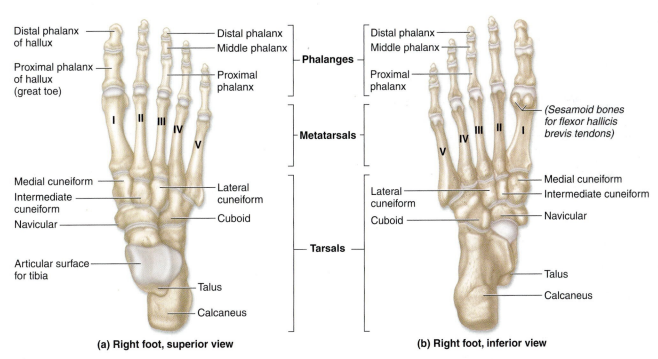

(a) Right foot, superior view

(b) Right foot, inferior view

Figure 1-4 Bones of the foot, inferior and superior views.

Major Bones of the Body

There are 206 bones in the human body: 80 in the axial skeleton and 126 in the appendicular skeleton. (See Figure 1-5 and Figure 1-6.) See Tables 1-3 and 1-4.

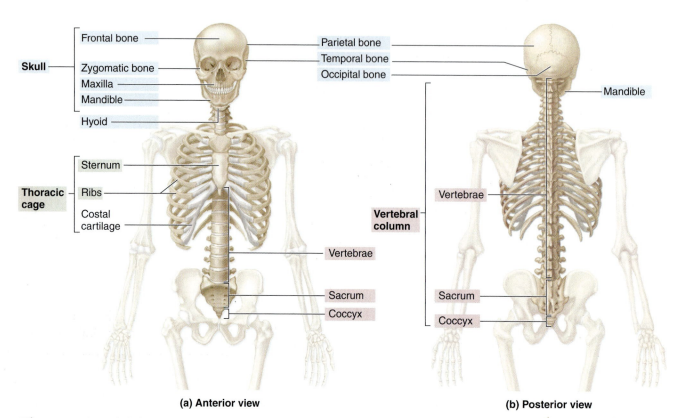

(a) Anterior view   **(b) Posterior view**

Figure 1-5 Axial skeleton.

TABLE 1-3	
At a Glance: Bones of the Axial Skeleton	
Skull (29)	Cranial bones (8): frontal (1), parietal (2), temporal (2), occipital (1), sphenoid (1), ethmoid (1)
	Facial bones (14): zygomatic (2), lacrimal (2), nasal (2), vomer (1), inferior nasal conchae (2), palatine (2), maxillae (2), mandible (1)
	Auditory ossicles: malleus (2), incus (2), stapes (2), hyoid (1)
Vertebral Column (26)	Vertebrae (24): cervical (7), thoracic (12), lumbar (5)
	Sacrum (1 bone of 3–5 fused)
	Coccyx (1 bone of 3 fused)
Thoracic Cage (25)	Sternum (1)
	Ribs (24)

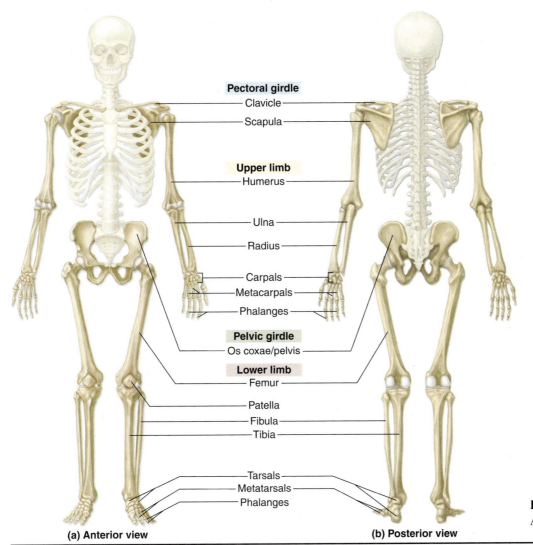

Pectoral girdle
Clavicle
Scapula

Upper limb
Humerus

Ulna

Radius

Carpals
Metacarpals
Phalanges

Pelvic girdle
Os coxae/pelvis

Lower limb
Femur

Patella
Fibula
Tibia

Tarsals
Metatarsals
Phalanges

(a) Anterior view

(b) Posterior view

Figure 1-6
Appendicular skeleton.

TABLE 1-4

At a Glance: Bones of the Appendicular Skeleton

Pectoral girdles (2 bones per each girdle, 4 bones total)	Clavicle (2) Scapula (2)
Upper limbs (30 bones per each upper limb, 60 bones total)	Humerus (2) Radius (2) Ulna (2) Carpals (16): scaphoid (2), lunate (2), triquetrum (2), pisiform (2), trapezium (2), trapezoid (2), capitate (2), hamate (2) Metacarpals (10) Phalanges (28) Proximal phalanx (10), middle phalanx (8), distal phalanx (10)
Pelvic girdles (1 bone per each girdle, 2 bones total)	Ossa coxae (2) Made up of Ilium (1), ishcium (1), pubis (1)
Lower limbs (30 bones per each lower limb, 60 bones total)	Femur (2) Patella (2) Tibia (2) Fibula (2) Tarsals (14): calcaneus (2), talus (2), navicular (2), cuboid (2), medial cuneiform (2), intermediate cuneiform (2), lateral cuneiform (2) Metatarsals (10) Phalanges (28) Proximal phalanx (10), middle phalanx (8), distal phalanx (10)

TABLE 1-5

At a Glance: Types of Muscle Fibers

Pattern of Muscle Fiber	Gross Appearance
Circular: Fibers arranged concentrically around an opening. Functions as a sphincter to close a passageway or opening (e.g., orbits, mouth, anus). *Example: Orbicularis oris*	Orbicularis oris
Convergent: Triangular muscle with common attachment site. The direction of pull can be changed; it does not pull as hard as an equal-sized parallel muscle. *Example: Pectoralis major*	Pectoralis major
Parallel: Fascicles are parallel to the long axis of the muscle. The body of the muscle increases in diameter with contraction. It is a high endurance muscle, but is not very strong. *Example: Rectus abdominis or sartorius*	Rectus abdominis
Pennate: The muscle body has one or more tendons; the fascicles are at an oblique angle to the tendon. This type of muscle pulls harder than a parallel muscle of equal size. Unipennate: These have all the muscle fibers on the same side of the tendon (e.g., extensor digitorum). Bipennate: These have muscle fibers on both sides of the tendon (e.g., rectus femoris). Multipennate: These muscles have tendons that branch within the muscle (e.g., deltoid).	Unipennate (extensor digitorum) Bipennate (rectus femoris) Multipennate (deltoid)

The Muscular System

FUNCTION: The muscular system provides the ability for movement, heat production, posture, and support. Several different muscle fiber patterns help define our muscles. See Table 1-5. Tendons attach muscle to bone.

Contraction: Contraction is shortening or tightening of a muscle. See Table 1-6. Skeletal muscles require actin, myosin, calcium, adenosine triphosphate (ATP), and neurotransmitters to contract. See Figure 1-7.

Sliding Filament Theory: The Sliding Filament Theory is a theory that explains muscular contractions. It states that if there is enough ATP, the myosin will attach to the actin and make the actin "slide" over each other, thus pulling the muscle fibers towards the center.

TABLE 1-6

At a Glance: Muscle Contraction

Components of a Muscle Contraction	Description
Actin	Small thin myofilaments
Myosin	Long thick myofilaments
Motor unit	One motor neuron and the muscle fibers it innervates
All or None Principle	States that a motor unit will either activate fully to 100%, or not activate at all (0%). The force of a contraction depends on how many motor units activate.

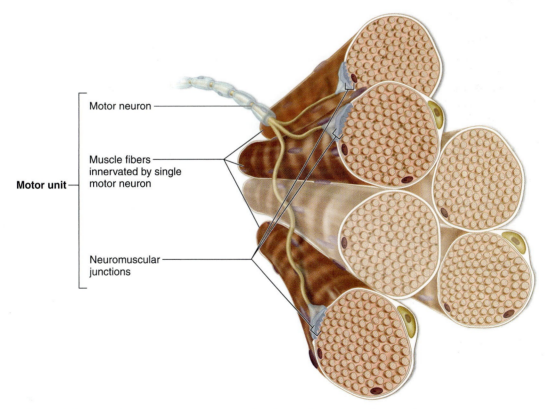

Figure 1-7 Muscle fibers within a motor unit may be distributed throughout the muscle.

The Nervous System

FUNCTION: Allows communication within the body (sensory and motor). There are two major divisions of the nervous system—the *central nervous system* and the *peripheral nervous system*.

Central Nervous System (CNS)

The central nervous system consists of the brain and spinal cord. The brain consists of four main parts: the cerebrum, cerebellum, diencephalon, and the brain stem. See Figure 1-8.

Meninges: The three layers that surround and protect the CNS are called the meninges. The *dura mater* is the thickest and most external layer. The *arachnoid* layer is web-like and provides space for the cerebrospinal fluid to circulate and cushion support. The *pia mater* is the softer, innermost layer. It is vascular and supplies nutrients to the brain.

Cerebrospinal fluid: This is a clear liquid that helps to cushion the brain and spinal cord. It also provides nutrients to the central nervous system.

Cerebrum: The cerebrum is the superior part of the brain, making up eighty-nine percent (89%) of the total brain mass. The right hemisphere (creativity) contains the sensory and motor pathways for the left side of the body. The left hemisphere (logic, science, languages, and verbal ideas) contains the sensory and motor pathways for the right side of the body. See Table 1-7.

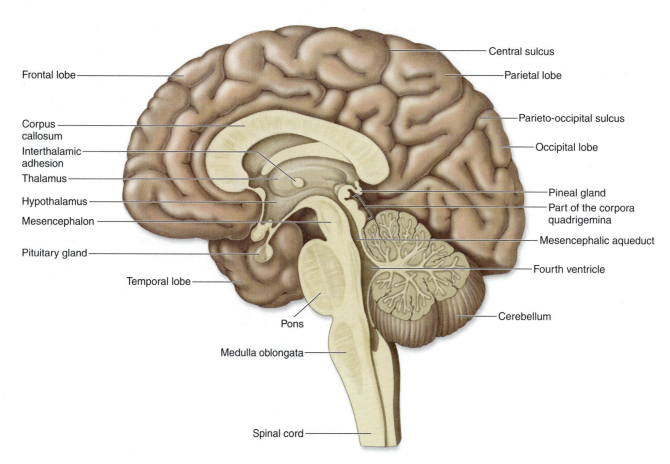

Figure 1-8 The sagittal view of the brain.

TABLE 1-7

At a Glance: Parts of the Brain and Their Functions

Brain	Function
Cerebrum	Right side: Creativity Left side: Logic, science, languages, verbal ideas
Cerebellum	Controls muscle tone, coordinates skeletal muscles and balance, and controls fine and gross motor movements
Diencephalon	Provides the relay and switching centers for some sensory and motor pathways and for control of visceral activities. Contains the thalamus and hypothalamus.
Brainstem	Contains three parts: Midbrain, pons, and medulla oblongata

Cerebellum: This is the second largest structure of the brain. It is found posterior and inferior to the cerebrum. The cerebellum coordinates and fine-tunes skeletal muscle movements. It also ensures that skeletal muscle contractions follow the correct pattern leading to smooth, coordinated movements. It also helps us to adjust skeletal muscle activity to help maintain equilibrium and posture.

Diencephalon: The diencephalon is often referred to as the "in-between brain." It provides the relay and switching centers for some sensory and motor pathways and for control of visceral activities.

- **Thalamus**: The thalamus sorts out and relays incoming sensory stimuli.

- **Hypothalamus:** The hypothalamus controls the pituitary gland and regulates water, electrolytes, balance, hunger, body temperature, sleep, sexual response, and emotions.

Brainstem: The brainstem interconnects many nervous pathways and contains three parts. See Table 1-8.

- **Midbrain**: This area is responsible for visual and auditory reflexes.
- **Pons**: This section of the brainstem is the center for autonomic respiration and acts as a bridge from the spine to the rest of the brain.
- **Medulla oblongata**: This area is the cardiac control center, vasomotor center, and respiratory center.

TABLE 1-8

At a Glance: Parts of the Brainstem and Diencephalon and Their Functions

Part of Diencephalon	Function
Thalamus	Relay station and interpretation center of the brain for all sensory impulses except olfactory
Hypothalamus	Governs homeostatic functions such as endocrine system and autonomic system
Part of Brainstem	**Function**
Midbrain	Houses voluntary motor tracts descending from the cerebral cortex to the spinal cord
Pons	Relays messages from the cerebral cortex to the spinal cord
Medulla oblongata	Respiratory center, cardiac center, vasomotor center. Also controls gastric secretions and reflexes

Peripheral Nervous System (PNS)

The peripheral nervous system contains all other nerves except the brain and spinal cord (cranial nerves and spinal nerves). See Figure 1-9. It is made up of two further divisions: the *somatic* and the *autonomic* systems.

Somatic nervous system: The part of the peripheral nervous system that controls skeletal muscles and their contractions.

Autonomic nervous system: The part of the peripheral nervous system that controls smooth muscle, cardiac muscle, internal organs, and glands. Within this system is the following:

- *Sympathetic nervous system* (fight or flight)
- *Parasympathetic nervous system* (rest and digest)

> **Memory Helper**
>
> The sympathetic system speeds us up, while the *para*sympathetic system is the *para*chute that slows us down.

Nerves that make up the PNS include the twelve cranial nerves and the nerves going to various muscles of the body. Let's take a look at the cranial nerves.

Cranial nerves: There are twelve pairs of cranial nerves, each designated by a name and a Roman numeral. Most cranial nerves are *mixed,* each consisting of both sensory and motor fibers. The cell bodies of the motor fibers are situated within the brain. The cell bodies of sensory fibers are located (for the most part) just outside the brain where they cluster together into a *ganglion.* See Table 1-9.

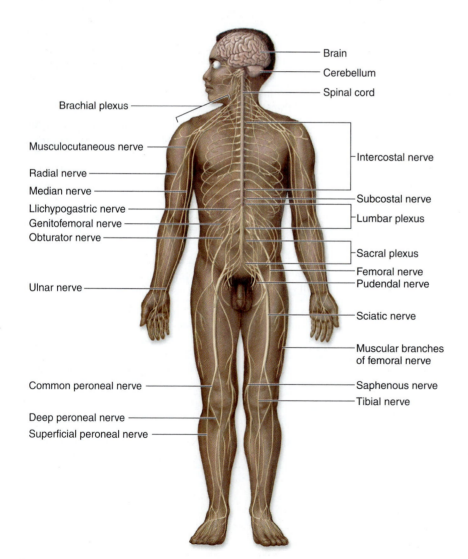

Figure 1-9 The peripheral nerves of the body.

> **Memory Helper**
>
> Mnemonic Device to Remember Cranial Nerves:
> Oh—Olfactory
> Oh—Optic
> Oh—Oculomotor
> To—Trochlear
> Touch—Trigeminal
> And—Abducens
> Feel—Facial
> Very—Vestibulocochlear
> Green—Glossopharyngeal
> Veggies—Vagus
> Ah—Accessory
> Ha—Hypoglossal

TABLE 1-9

At a Glance: The Cranial Nerves

I Olfactory nerves (sensory):	There are actually many tiny olfactory nerves, each originating in the roof of the nasal cavity and terminating in the olfactory bulb. The olfactory nerves conduct impulses from the nasal cavity to the olfactory area of the cerebral cortex, which interprets these impulses as *smell*.
II Optic nerve (sensory):	The fibers of the optic nerve originate in the retina (back of the eye). From there, the fibers conduct impulses to the midbrain. From the midbrain, the impulses are relayed to the visual area of the cerebral cortex where the impulses are interpreted as *sight*.
III Oculomotor nerve (mixed):	The sensory and motor fibers of this nerve supply the muscles that produce *movements of the eye ball*, as well as the eye lid muscles. It also supplies the iris (the sphincter muscle through which light enters the eye) and the ciliary muscles, which change the shape of the lens to accommodate for near and far vision. Damage to this nerve may result in double vision, dilated pupils, blurred vision, and droopy eyelids (ptosis).
IV Trochlear nerve (mixed):	This is the smallest of the cranial nerves. Its sensory and motor fibers supply the superior oblique muscles for *oblique eye movements*.
V Trigeminal nerve (mixed):	This is the largest of the cranial nerves. It supplies the tissues of the face, eyes, nasal cavity, and mouth. Sensory fibers conduct impulses for touch, heat, cold, and pain (including tooth pain). Motor fibers supply the chewing muscles. Its name is taken from the fact that it consists of three main branches: the ophthalmic nerve (supplies the scalp, eyes, outer nose, and nasal cavity), the *maxillary* nerve (supplies the nasal cavity, palate, and upper teeth), and the *mandibular* nerve (supplies the lower jaw and teeth).
VI Abducens nerve (mixed):	The sensory and motor fibers of this nerve supply the lateral rectus muscles for *lateral eye movements*.
VII Facial nerve (mixed):	Sensory fibers conduct impulses from the *taste buds* on the anterior two-thirds of the tongue. Motor fibers supply the *facial muscles.* Bell's palsy is a dysfunction of the facial nerve. The muscles are paralyzed on one side of the face, and the person loses sensation on that side of the face, the lower eyelid droops, the corner of the mouth sags, there is partial loss of taste, and the eyes tear constantly. The cause is unknown, symptoms could disappear spontaneously, and massage can help.
VIII Vestibulocochlear nerve (sensory):	Also known as the statoacoustic nerve and *auditory nerve.* It originates in the ear. It has two portions: the *vestibular* portion conducts impulses which the brain uses to get a sense of balance. The *cochlear* portion carries impulses to the auditory area of the cerebral cortex which interprets the impulses as "sound." Damage to this nerve results in impaired hearing (nerve deafness), dizziness, and nausea.
IX Glossopharyngeal nerve (mixed):	This nerve supplies the back of the tongue (glosso) and the throat (pharynx). Sensory fibers provide general sensation for these areas as well as taste information from the back of the tongue. Sensory fibers originating from the carotid artery gives the brain information about blood pressure. Motor fibers supply swallowing muscles of the throat. Damage to this nerve results in loss of gag reflex and impaired ability to swallow and taste (sour and bitter).
X Vagus nerve (mixed):	This nerve supplies most of the visceral organs in the thoracic and abdominopelvic cavity. Damage results in hoarseness, loss of voice, difficulty in swallowing, and impaired digestion. Innervates smooth muscle of heart and lungs.
XI Accessory nerve (motor):	Motor fibers supply the sternocleidomastoid muscle (SCM), traps, and swallowing muscles. Damage may result in turning of the head to one side (SCM) and impaired ability to shrug shoulder (traps).
XII Hypoglossal nerve (motor):	Motor fibers supply muscles of the tongue. Damage results in impaired ability to speak and swallow.

Trigeminal neuralgia: (*neuro = nerve; algia = pain*) Also known as *tic douloureux*, it is among the most severely painful conditions that exist. It is caused by inflammation of the trigeminal nerve. The pain may last for a few seconds or a few minutes, but it may occur many times during the day. It may be triggered by the slightest amount of stimulation, such as brushing the teeth or a puff of air hitting the face. Severing of the nerve just proximal to its ganglion treats the most severe cases.

The peripheral nerves branch off from the spinal nerves to innervate specific muscles. See Tables 1-10 and 1-11.

Special Senses

The peripheral nervous system also includes special senses. The special senses are sight, smell, hearing, taste, and position. The body has muscle spindles and golgi tendons to help us with body position (*proprioception*).

Proprioception: Proprioception is the ability to tell where our body or parts are without having to look.

For example, if you close your eyes and hold your arm up at shoulder level, you know it is at shoulder level without having to look.

Muscle spindles: Muscles spindles help our body protect itself from over-stretching. Remember reaching for something that was just out of reach? Your muscles may have cramped a little to let you know they cannot go that far, thanks to those muscle spindles.

Golgi tendons: The Golgi tendons are nerve endings located within tendons near a muscle-tendon junction. They help us from over-contracting by sending signals to the interneurons in the spinal cord which in turn inhibit the actions of the motor neurons. This allows the muscle to relax, thus protecting the muscle and tendon from excessive tension damage. Remember the last time you tried to pick up a box that weighed too much? Your muscles cramped or tensed so that you could not lift it and hurt yourself, thanks to those Golgi tendons. This is overridden in fight or flight, such as the small person who is miraculously able to lift the car off the person trapped underneath.

Stretch reflex: The stretch reflex is the utilization of both Golgi tendons and muscle spindles to help us stretch. By holding our stretches for ten seconds or longer, we are telling the Golgi tendons they are not needed, so the muscle spindles can take over and help the muscles to elongate and let us know how far we can stretch without tearing. If we do not hold our stretches long enough, the Golgi tendons think we are exercising; therefore, they think they must activate. When they activate, they tighten our muscles to prevent us from over-contracting.

TABLE 1-10

At a Glance: Spinal Nerves

Spinal Nerves	Number of Pairs
Cervical nerves (C1–C8)	8 pair
Thoracic nerves (T1–T12)	12 pair
Lumbar nerves (L1–L5)	5 pair
Sacral nerves (S1–S5)	5 pair
Coccygeal (CX)	1 pair
Total Nerves	31 pairs

TABLE 1-11

At a Glance: Major Peripheral Nerves and the Muscle Innervations

Nerve	Muscle
Phrenic nerve	Diaphragm
Axillary nerve	Deltoid, teres minor
Musculocutaneous nerve	Anterior brachium
Median nerve	Anterior forearm, hand
Ulnar nerve	Medial anterior forearm, hand
Radial nerve	Posterior arm, posterior forearm
Femoral nerve	Anterior thigh
Obturator nerve	Medial thigh
Sciatic nerve	Posterior thigh
Tibial nerve	Posterior leg, plantar foot
Superficial peroneal nerve	Lateral leg
Deep peroneal nerve	Anterior leg, dorsal foot
Common peroneal nerve	Back of the knee (splits into deep and superficial nerves)

The Endocrine System

FUNCTION: The endocrine system secretes hormones that help to regulate homeostasis and body function. See Figure 1-10.

Pineal gland: The pineal gland is a tiny structure situated just above the thalamus in an area of the brain known as the *epithalamus*. The pineal gland produces a hormone called melatonin. In humans, the function of melatonin is not clear. It appears to play a role in maintaining day/night rhythms, and it also appears to inhibit the premature secretions of female hormones prior to puberty.

Pituitary gland: The pituitary gland hangs down from the hypothalamus and is housed within the sella turcica, a pocket on the floor of the cranium (sphenoid bone). Small as it is, this gland has earned the name "master gland of the body" because its hormones control the activity of other endocrine glands. However, it is by no means the absolute master. Its secretions are carefully regulated by the hypothalamus of the brain. Recall that the hypothalamus has within it control centers (nuclei) which monitor the condition of our internal environment. These control centers regulate the internal environment by (1) sending impulses through the autonomic system or (2) influencing the pituitary gland.

Thyroid gland: The thyroid gland is situated at the base of the neck. It secretes two hormones: *thyroxin* and *thyrocalcitonin*. Thyrocalcitonin decreases the level of calcium ions in the blood by causing the calcium to be absorbed by bone. Thyroxin has several functions:

- Stimulates growth in children (anabolism)
- Stimulates the breakdown of glucose for energy (catabolism)

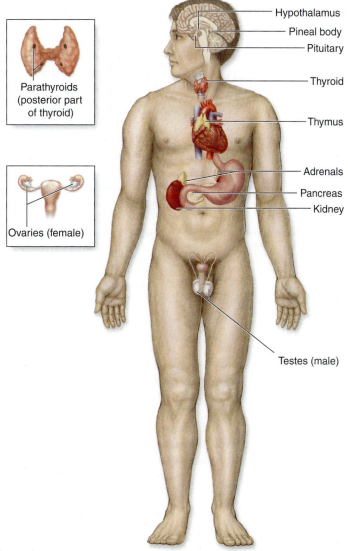

Parathyroids (posterior part of thyroid)

Ovaries (female)

Hypothalamus
Pineal body
Pituitary
Thyroid
Thymus
Adrenals
Pancreas
Kidney
Testes (male)

Figure 1-10 The endocrine system.

Hypothyroidism: This is a condition in which there is a lack of thyroxin in the blood. If this happens in the growth years, it results in mental retardation and dwarfism characterized by a large head and small limbs. Hypothyroidism after the growth years results in low metabolic rate, depression, fatigue, weight gain, and tendency to retain water, especially in the face.

Hyperthyroidism: Hyperthyroidism is due to over-secretion of thyroxin characterized by irritability, weight loss, enlarged thyroid gland (goiter), and bulging eyes (exophthalmia).

Parathyroid glands: Four small nodules found on the back of the thyroid gland. (Some people may have as few as two or as many as six.) These glands produce *parathyroid hormone* (PTH), which increases blood calcium by causing the release of calcium from bone.

Thymus: The thymus is located behind the sternum. It is large in children and diminishes in size throughout adulthood. The hormones of the thymus are essential to the development of the immune system and T-cells.

Adrenal glands: Each of the two adrenal glands is situated on the superior surface of one kidney. Each gland consists of an outer cortex and an inner medulla.

Two hormones produced by the adrenal medulla are *adrenaline* (epinephrine) and *noradrenaline* (norepinephrine). They are both produced from the amino acid tyrosine. Both hormones seem to affect the body in the same manner as the sympathetic system. In other words, they increase heart rate and respiration. Adrenaline is the more potent of the two.

The Cardiovascular System

FUNCTION: Allows the body to receive nourishment via the blood as well as transports waste for removal by other organs. The cardiovascular system consists of the heart, arteries, veins, and capillaries. Blood is made of plasma (55%) which is composed of water, salts, nutrients, hormones, and plasma proteins. Formed elements make up 45% of blood and include red blood cells, white blood cells, and platelets.

Heart: The heart is a pump that drives blood through the blood vessels. It has three layers of muscle: the *endocardium*, the *myocardium*, and the *pericardium*. See Table 1-12.

TABLE 1-12

At a Glance: Layers of the Heart Muscle and Their Locations

Layer of the Heart	Location
Endocardium	The thin membrane lining the inner wall of the heart
Myocardium	The thick middle layer composed of cardiac muscle tissue
Pericardium	The thin membrane covering the outer side of the heart

Arteries: Arteries are blood vessels that carry blood away from the heart. All arteries have oxygenated blood in them with the exception of the pulmonary artery which has deoxygenated blood.

Veins: These blood vessels carry blood towards the heart. All veins in the body have deoxygenated blood with the exception of the pulmonary vein which has oxygenated blood.

Capillaries: Capillaries are microscopic blood vessels where the exchange of oxygen into the tissue takes place.

Endocarditis: This is an inflammation of the inner layer of the heart.

Pericarditis: This is an inflammation of the outer layer of the heart.

Chambers of the heart: The four chambers of the heart are the *right atrium, left atrium, right ventricle,* and *left ventricle.* See Figure 1-11.

Cardiac blood supply: Four large blood vessels supply the heart. The *superior vena cava* and the *inferior vena cava* are the two main veins that collect blood from the body and channel it to the heart. The *pulmonary artery* channels blood away from the heart to the lungs. The *pulmonary veins* channel blood from the lungs to the heart. The *aorta* is the largest artery in the body. It conducts blood from the heart to the body. See Table 1-13.

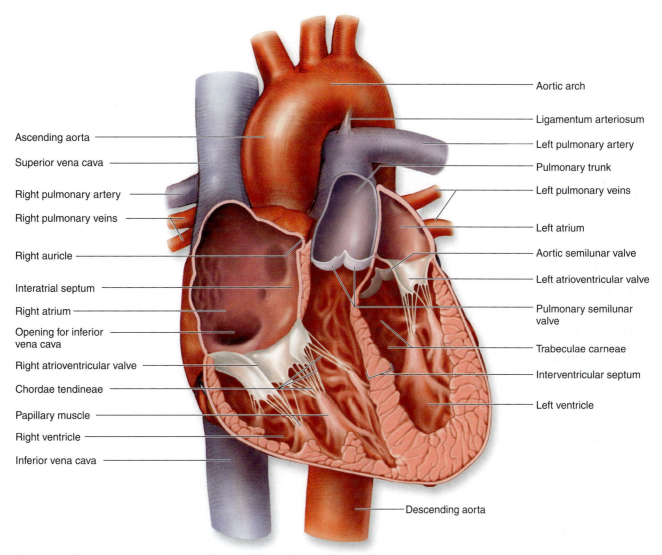

Aortic arch

Ligamentum arteriosum

Left pulmonary artery

Pulmonary trunk

Left pulmonary veins

Left atrium

Aortic semilunar valve

Left atrioventricular valve

Pulmonary semilunar valve

Trabeculae carneae

Interventricular septum

Left ventricle

Ascending aorta

Superior vena cava

Right pulmonary artery

Right pulmonary veins

Right auricle

Interatrial septum

Right atrium

Opening for inferior vena cava

Right atrioventricular valve

Chordae tendineae

Papillary muscle

Right ventricle

Inferior vena cava

Descending aorta

Figure 1-11 Anatomy of the heart.

TABLE 1-13

At a Glance: Vessels of the Heart and Their Functions

Heart Vessel	Purpose
Vena cavas (inferior and superior)	Main veins that return blood to the heart
Pulmonary artery	The artery leading from the right ventricle of the heart to the lungs
Pulmonary vein	Returns blood from the lungs to the left atrium of the heart

TABLE 1-14

At a Glance: Valves of the Heart and Their Locations

Heart Valve	Location
Right atrio-ventricular valve (tricuspid valve)	Between the right atrium and right ventricle
Left atrio-ventricular valve (mitral valve)	Between the left atrium and left ventricle
Pulmonary semilunar valve	Between the right ventricle and the pulmonary artery
Aortic semilunar valve	Between the left ventricle and the aorta

Cardiac valves: Four valves keep the blood flowing in the proper direction through the heart. See Table 1-14.

1. The *right atrio-ventricular* (AV) *valve* (aka: *tricuspid valve*) is the trap door between the right atrium and the right ventricle. It is also called the tricuspid valve because it is composed of three flaps of tissue.
2. The *left atrio-ventricular valve* (aka: *mitral valve*) is the trap door between the left atrium and the left ventricle. It is also called the bicuspid valve because it is composed of two flaps of tissue. The early anatomists called it the mitral valve because they imagined that its two flaps of tissue resembled the fancy hat (mitre) worn by bishops.

3. The *pulmonary semilunar valve* is the valve situated between the right ventricle and the pulmonary artery.
4. The *aortic semilunar* valve is the valve situated between the left ventricle and the aorta.

Cardiac blood flow: The heart is two pumps in one. The right side of the heart receives oxygen-depleted blood from the body in general and pumps it to the lungs. The left side of the heart receives the freshly oxygenated blood from the lungs and propels it through the body in general (Figure 1-12). Deoxygenated blood flows from the body through the vena cavas into the right atrium. Then blood flows

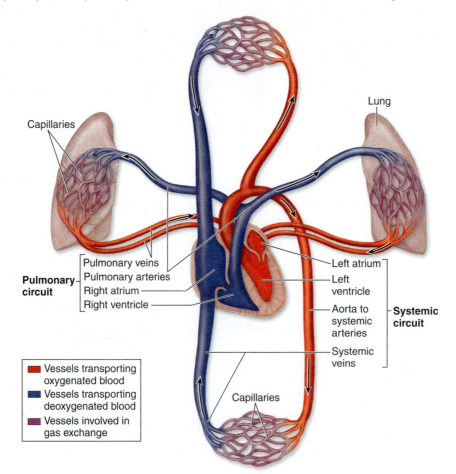

Figure 1-12 Blood flow. The right ventricle forces blood to the lungs; the left ventricle forces blood to the rest of the body.

through the AV valve into the right ventricle, through the pulmonary artery, to the lungs. Once in the lungs, the blood is filled with oxygen. The blood flows back to the heart via the pulmonary vein and goes into the left atrium, through the mitral valve, and into the left ventricle. The left ventricle pumps the blood through the aorta where the newly oxygenated blood can get to the rest of the body.

Cardiac circulation: The heart maintains two circulatory pathways, the pulmonary circulation and systemic circulation. See Table 1-15. *Pulmonary circulation* is the circulation of the blood from the heart to the lungs and back to the heart. *Systemic circulation* may be summarized as follows: the left ventricle contracts and sends the blood surging through the aorta. The aorta branches off into a series of progressively smaller arteries. The smallest arteries are microscopic vessels called arterioles which send blood into the capillaries. As the blood flows through the capillaries, nutrients and oxygen filter out through the walls of the capillaries and become part of the tissue. In this manner, the cells of the body are nourished. Meanwhile carbon dioxide, ammonia, and other cellular waste products diffuse into the capillaries. The capillaries channel the blood into tiny veins called venules. These collect into a series of progressively larger and larger veins. All the veins in systemic circulation collect into the superior and inferior vena cavas which channels the blood back into the right atrium of the heart. The skeletal muscle and respiratory pumping action helps boost venous return.

Arteriosclerosis: Also known as hardening of the arteries, this condition is due to calcium deposits on the walls of arteries.

Atherosclerosis: This is a condition in which fatty material becomes deposited on the walls of arteries, thus narrowing the passageway for blood.

Aneurysm: This is a ballooning out of the arterial wall. The ballooned arteries are weaker than the rest of the area and are more vulnerable to rupturing, especially if the blood pressure is abnormally high.

Blood pressure: The force that blood exerts on the walls of blood vessels is called blood pressure. Blood pressure is greatest as it leaves the heart and surges through the large arteries. It drops steadily as it flows through the smaller arteries, capillaries, small veins, and large veins. It is lowest in the largest veins, just before it enters the heart.

Major Arterial Roots

Arterial roots accompany nerve roots into the spinal cord. Major roots include the following:

- Head—common carotid arteries
- Upper extremities—subclavian arteries → axillary arteries → brachial arteries → radial and ulnar arteries
- Lower extremities—common iliac arteries → external iliac arteries → femoral arteries

In addition, these major arterial roots contain major pulse points in the body. Because of the need for blood flow to organs in muscles, these pulse points are also generally endangerment sites for massage. See Table 1-16.

TABLE 1-16

At a Glance: Pulse Points

Pulse Point	Location
Temporal artery	Anterior and slightly superior to the temporomandibular joint (TMJ)
Common carotid	Medial to the SCM
Axillary	Axilla
Brachial	Medial to biceps brachii
Radial	Thumb side of anterior wrist
Ulnar	Medial anterior wrist
Abdominal aorta	Between xiphoid and navel, just to left of midline
Femoral	Just below inguinal ligament in proximal anterior thigh
Popliteal	Popliteal region
Posterior tibial	Posterior to medial malleolus
Dorsal pedis	Anterior to medial malleolus

TABLE 1-15

At a Glance: Types of Circulation

Type of Circulation	Circulatory Pathway
Pulmonary circulation	From the heart to the lungs and back
Systemic circulation	From the heart to the rest of the body and back

TABLE 1-17

At a Glance: Pathologies of Blood Vessels

Condition	Definition
Phlebitis	Inflammation of a vein
Thrombophlebitis	A blood clot from the result of phlebitis
Thrombus	A clot in a non-traumatized blood vessel
Embolus	A moving blood clot

Pathologies of Blood Vessels

Varicose veins: This is an abnormal distention of veins, usually due to sluggish circulation. Varicosities are most common in the lower extremity.

Hemorrhoids: These are varicosities in the veins of the anus.

Phlebitis: Phlebitis is inflammation of a vein. It is accompanied by redness of the overlying skin and throbbing pain. It is usually caused by bacterial infection or local trauma. See Table 1-17.

Thrombophlebitis: This is blood clotting in the affected vein. Severe cases of phlebitis may progress to this condition. The danger of thrombophlebitis is that the thrombus may become dislodged.

Thrombus: Thrombus is a clot that develops in a non-traumatized blood vessel.

Embolus: An embolus is a moving clot which may later become lodged in a small artery and obstruct blood flow to a vital organ. An embolus lodged in a small artery in the brain may result in a stroke. An embolus lodged in the heart or lungs may be fatal.

The Lymph System

FUNCTION: Helps the body with immunity, drains fluids from tissues, and filters waste via the lymph. The lymph vascular system consists of lymph vessels and a number of lymphatic organs. These organs are lymph nodes, tonsils, spleen, and thymus. The movement of lymph is primarily done by muscular movement and by gravity.

Lymph vessels: The lymph vessels of the body are essentially a system of filters that drain off excess tissue fluid and channel it back to the blood stream from whence it came. The smallest lymph vessels are the blind-ended lymph capillaries which absorb excess tissue fluid. Once the fluid enters the lymph capillaries, it is called "lymph." The lymph capillaries merge into a series of progressively larger lymph vessels which follow a similar course as the veins, and like the veins, they have valves which keep the lymph flowing in one direction.

Lymphatic ducts: All the lymph vessels in the body drain into two main lymphatic ducts which are situated in the thoracic cavity. The left and right thoracic ducts drain into the left and right subclavian veins. Massage is excellent for cleaning out stagnant tissue fluid and lymph.

Lymph nodes: Lymph nodes are sometimes erroneously called lymph glands. If lymph vessels of the body may be likened to sewer pipes, the lymph nodes may be compared to the sewage processing centers. Lymph nodes are pea-sized pellets situated along the course of lymph vessels. Each is covered with connective tissue and is filled with macrophages. As the lymph passes through the node, the macrophages engulf the debris and bacteria in the lymph. The nodes also produce *lymphocytes* and *monocytes*.

Lymphocytes: There are three types of lymphocytes. *T-lymphocytes* help to recognize antigens and attack foreign cells to reduce threats by pathogens. *B-lymphocytes* contain antigen receptors that respond to one particular antigen and cause the production of antibodies to respond to that particular antigen. NK (natural killer) cells are the third type. These kill a wide variety of infected or cancerous cells. They respond to multiple antigens.

Tonsils: Tonsils are small lymphatic organs located in the throat. There are three pairs of tonsils:

1. Pharyngeal tonsils located in the upper throat;
2. Palatine tonsils next to the soft palate; and
3. Lingual tonsils at the base of the tongue.

Like lymph nodes, they are centers for the generation of lymphocytes. They also play a role in policing the tissues of the throat.

Tonsillectomy: The removal of tonsils is performed when the organ becomes so infected and enlarged that it interferes with the passage of food and air. The palatine tonsils are usually removed.

Adenoids: Adenoids are enlarged pharyngeal tonsils.

Thymus: The thymus is a two-lobed organ situated in the upper thoracic cavity behind the sternum about one-half to one inch below the sternal ridge. It is large in children and decreases in size (relative to the rest of the body) as the individual ages. It produces hormones that seem to be essential for the maturation of certain lymphocytes (T-lymphocytes).

Spleen: The spleen is a reddish-brown organ located just under the diaphragm, posterior and lateral to the stomach. It contains macrophages which engulf worn-out blood cells and bacteria. The spleen also produces lymphocytes and monocytes. In mononucleosis, the spleen becomes enlarged because it's busy producing large amounts of monocytes. The spleen also stores about 200 milliliters of whole blood which may be ejected into the blood stream during severe hemorrhage.

The Urinary System

FUNCTION: To remove waste and excess water from the body and excess chemicals from the blood.

Kidneys:

The kidneys are situated against the posterior wall of the trunk between T-12 and L-1 (bottom of the rib cage). See Figure 1-13. The right kidney is slightly lower than the left due to the crowding effect of the liver. Each kidney is shaped like a lima bean. The kidney is four to five inches long, two to three inches wide, and one inch thick. The hilum, a notch on the concave medial surface of the kidney, provides passage for the ureter, blood vessels, lymph vessels, and nerves that supply the kidney. Specific functions of the kidneys include the following:

- Filtration of blood to remove waste, excess salts, and toxins
- Production of urine to excrete unwanted materials
- Maintenance of water balance for the body
- Regulation of acid–base balance
- Production of hormones
- Maintenance of blood pressure

Nephrons: Nephrons are the structural and functional unit of the kidney. They are located in the cortex of the kidney and do the job of filtering and removing waste from the blood and collecting it as urine.

Ureters: These are the tubes that transfer urine from the kidneys to the bladder.

Urethra: This is the canal that allows for transfer of urine from the bladder for excretion.

Bladder: The bladder is a muscular organ for storage of urine. It is located on the floor of the pelvic cavity just posterior to the pubic bone.

Urine formation occurs in three steps:

1. *Glomerular filtration* is filtration of fluid out of the capillaries and into the nephron. The driving force for this process is blood pressure.
2. *Tubular reabsorption* is the reabsorption of chemicals from the nephron back to the blood.
3. *Tubular secretion* is the addition of specific chemicals (potassium ions, hydrogen ions, ammonia, and drugs) to the fluid as it flows through the last part of the nephron. By the time the fluid reaches the end of the nephron and enters the collecting tubule, it is called urine.

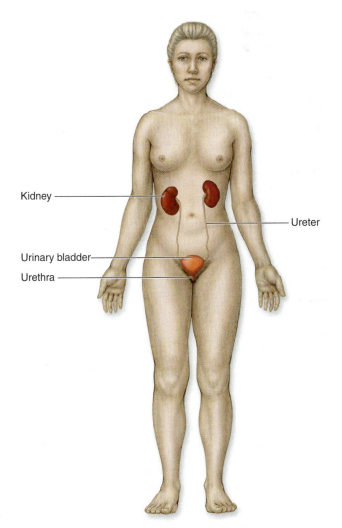

Figure 1-13 The urinary system.

The Respiratory System

FUNCTION: The respiratory system facilitates the exchange of gases from the air into the body and bloodstream. See Figure 1-14. The respiratory system contains several components.

Sinuses: The sinuses (frontal, maxillary, and sphenoidal) are hollow spaces in the bones of the head. Small openings connect them to the nose. The functions they serve include helping to regulate the temperature and humidity of air breathed in, as well as lightening the bone structure of the head and giving resonance to the voice.

Nose: The nose (nasal cavity) is the preferred entrance for outside air into the respiratory system. It helps to warm and moisten the air as it enters the body. The hairs that line the wall of the nose are part of the air-cleaning system, helping to trap dust and mucus for removal.

Mouth: Air also enters through the mouth (oral cavity), especially in people who have a mouth-breathing habit or whose nasal passages may be temporarily obstructed, as by a cold or during heavy exercise. The air is not filtered like it is through the nose; therefore, in non-labored breathing, nose breathing is best.

Pharynx: The pharynx is also called the throat. The pharynx collects incoming air from the nose and mouth and passes it downward to the larynx.

Epiglottis: The epiglottis is a flap of tissue that guards the entrance to the laryngeal opening, closing when anything is swallowed that should go into the esophagus and stomach.

Larynx: The larynx is the organ of voice; it contains the vocal cords. Air moving in and out creates voice sounds.

Esophagus: This is the passage leading from the mouth and throat to the stomach.

Trachea: The trachea is the passage leading from the throat (pharynx) to the lungs. The windpipe divides into the two main bronchial tubes, one for each lung, which subdivide into each lobe of the lungs. These, in turn, subdivide further.

Bronchial tubes: The right lung is divided into three *lobes,* or sections; the left lung is divided into two lobes or sections. Each lobe is like a balloon filled with sponge-like tissue. Air moves in and out through one opening—a branch of the bronchial tube.

Pleura: These are the two membranes, actually one continuous membrane folded on itself, that surround

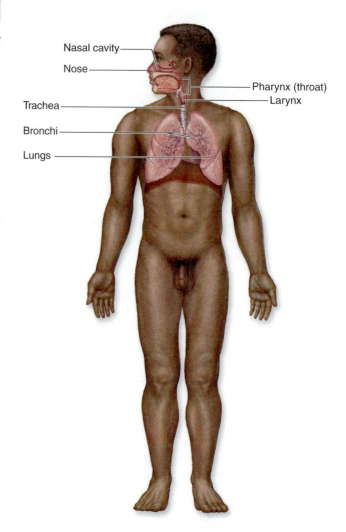

Figure 1-14 The respiratory system.

each lobe of the lungs and separate the lungs from the chest wall.

Diaphragm: This is the strong wall of muscle that separates the chest cavity from the abdominal cavity. By moving downward, it creates suction in the chest to draw in air and expand the lungs.

Bronchioles: Bronchioles are the smallest subdivisions of the bronchial tubes, at the end of which are the air sacs or alveoli (plural of alveolus).

Alveoli: These are the very small air sacs where oxygen goes before it is absorbed into the blood stream. The respiratory system can further be divided into upper and lower structures. See Table 1-18.

TABLE 1-18

At a Glance: Structures of the Upper and Lower Respiratory System

Upper Respiratory Structures	Lower Respiratory Structures
Nasal cavity	Larynx
Paranasal sinuses	Trachea
Pharynx	Bronchi
	Bronchioles
	Alveoli ducts and alveoli

Respiration: Respiration, in the broadest sense, refers to the exchange of gases between living cells and their environment. In humans, respiration involves three processes.

1. **Ventilation (breathing):** This is the exchange of gases between the atmosphere and lungs. It involves taking air into the lungs (inhalation) and expelling air from the lungs (exhalation). Inhalation is an active process meaning that it depends on the contraction of muscles (mostly the diaphragm). See Figure 1-15. Exhalation is normally a passive process because it happens as a consequence of the relaxation of the breathing muscles. However, we can produce forceful exhalation by contracting the abdominal muscles which pushes air out more forcefully than it would otherwise. Coughing, sneezing, and laughing are examples of forceful exhalation.

   The total amount of air that both lungs can hold is approximately 6000 ml. This is known as *total lung capacity.* However, in normal inhalation, we do not fill the lungs to capacity, and in normal exhalation, we certainly do not expel all the air from the lungs. The normal amount of air that is inhaled and exhaled in quiet breathing is about 500 ml; this is called the *tidal volume.* The largest volume of air that may be drawn in after the most powerful exhalation is called the *vital capacity,* which is about 5000 ml.

2. **External respiration:** The exchange of gases between the alveoli and the blood is external respiration. The alveoli are surrounded by a cluster of capillaries. As the blood flows through these capillaries, oxygen from the alveoli diffuses into the capillaries, and carbon dioxide diffuses from the capillaries into the alveoli.

3. **Internal respiration:** This is the exchange of gases between the blood and the body cells. It is essentially the reverse of what happens in the alveoli of the lungs.

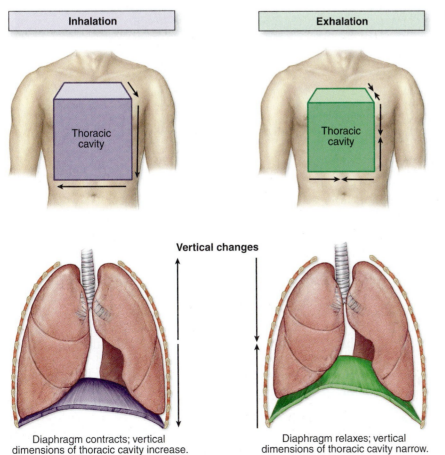

Figure 1-15 Movement of the diaphragm during respiration.

Inhalation

Thoracic cavity

Exhalation

Thoracic cavity

Vertical changes

Diaphragm contracts; vertical dimensions of thoracic cavity increase.

Diaphragm relaxes; vertical dimensions of thoracic cavity narrow.

The Gastrointestinal System

FUNCTION: The gastrointestinal system helps us to receive nutrients by taking in and digesting food as well as absorb water and remove waste. See Figure 1-16.

Teeth: The teeth are housed within alveoli, pocket-like hollows within the mandible and maxillae. Each of the thirty-two teeth has three sections: The *crown* is the visible section. The *root* is the part embedded in the alveoli. And the *neck* is the constricted portion between the crown and root. Teeth are not made of bone; although like bone, they are composed primarily of calcium phosphate. The bulk of the tooth is made of a harder-than-bone substance called *dentin*. The dentin of the root is covered by another hard substance called the cementum. The crown is covered by enamel, which is the hardest of the three.

Tongue: The tongue serves as an organ of taste, with taste buds scattered over its surface and concentrated toward the back of the tongue. In chewing, the tongue holds the food against the teeth; in swallowing, it moves the food back into the pharynx and then into the esophagus when the pressure of the tongue closes the opening of the trachea, or windpipe. It also acts, together with the lips, teeth, and hard palate, to form word sounds.

Salivary glands: On the floor of the mouth are three pairs of salivary glands. These glands secrete saliva which is channeled to the surface through ducts. Saliva is 99.5 percent water. The rest is salts, urea, uric acid, mucus, and enzymes. One of the enzymes is amylase which begins the digestion of complex carbohydrates (usually starch).

Esophagus: This is about ten inches long, spanning the distance between the pharynx and stomach. The opening between the stomach and esophagus is guarded by a ring of muscle called the cardiac sphincter, so named because of its close proximity to the heart. The cardiac sphincter is also called the gastroesophogeal sphincter.

Stomach: Situated just under the diaphragm on the left side of the abdominal cavity. The stomach has a capacity of about one and one-half liters, but when it is empty, it can shrink down to the size of a fist. The upper portion of the stomach is called the fundus, the middle portion is called the body, and the lower portion is called the pylorus. The latter has the pyloric

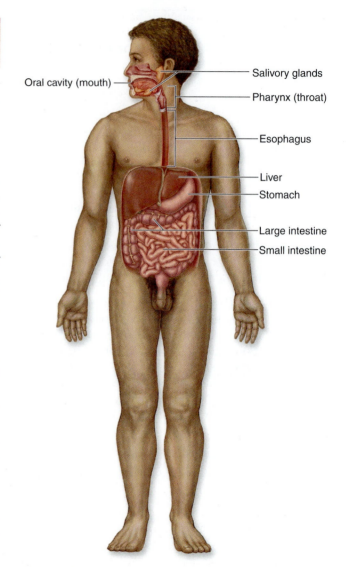

Figure 1-16 The gastrointestinal (digestive) system.

sphincter, a ring of muscle which guards the opening between the end of the stomach and the beginning of the small intestine.

Small intestine: The small intestine is a tube about 20 feet long and one inch wide. It is divided into three parts: The first ten inches are a C-shaped expanded portion called the *duodenum* which merges with the stomach. The next seven feet are called the *jejunum*. The last twelve feet are called the *ileum*, which merges with the large intestine. The small intestine is where most digestion and absorption takes place.

Large intestine: The large intestine is about five feet long and two to three inches wide. Its three parts are the *cecum, colon,* and *rectum.* The cecum is the first three to four inches which merges with the small intestines. The opening between the end of the small intestine and the beginning of the large intestine is guarded by the ileo-cecal valve. The very tip of the cecum has a squiggly tube called the vermiform appendix, which literally means "worm-like appendage."

Colon: The colon forms the bulk of the large intestine. It is divided into four parts: the *ascending colon,* the *transverse colon,* the *descending colon,* and the *sigmoid colon.* The last five to six inches of the large intestine is an expanded pouch called the rectum which opens to the outside via the anal canal. The external opening of the anal canal is called the anus.

Pancreas: The pancreas is a carrot-like organ situated just below the stomach. Its wide, medial end is tucked inside the "C" of the duodenum, and the pointed lateral end touches the spleen. Pockets of endocrine cells called the Islets of Langerhans produce glucagons and insulin hormones that regulate blood-sugar levels. The pancreas also aids in digestion of fats and proteins.

Liver: The liver is the largest internal organ in the human body and also one of the most important. It has many functions, among them the synthesis of proteins, immune and clotting factors, and oxygen and fat-carrying substances. Its chief digestive function is the secretion of bile, a solution critical to fat emulsion and absorption. The liver also removes excess glucose from circulation and stores it until it is needed. It converts excess amino acids into useful forms and filters drugs and poisons from the bloodstream, neutralizing them and excreting them in bile. The liver has two main lobes, located just under the diaphragm on the right side of the body. It can lose up to seventy-five percent of its tissue (to disease or surgery) without ceasing to function. The liver also does the following:

- Detoxifies the blood
- Prepares nutrients to be utilized by the body cells
- Produces most of the plasma proteins in the blood
- Stores iron, vitamin A, and glycogen
- Destroys old blood cells
- Produces cholesterol
- Changes some of the cholesterol into bile salts
- Produces bile

Gallbladder: The gallbladder is located under and is attached to the liver and serves as a reservoir for bile. As it is produced by the liver, bile passes to the gallbladder through a small tube called the cystic duct. The gallbladder's muscular walls absorb excess water and, when stimulated, contract to squirt concentrated bile through the biliary ducts and into the small intestine, where it aids in digestion.

The Reproductive System

FUNCTION: To allow for reproduction.

Genitalia: These are the reproductive organs of males and females.

Gonads: One of the two types of primary reproductive organs, ovaries (female) and testes (male).

Gamete: This is a cell with half the number of chromosomes. The other half of the chromosomes will come from the male gamete which is the spermatozoan.

The Male Reproductive System

Testis/testes: This is the male gonad. The two testes are normally situated in the scrotum and produce sperm cells and male sex hormones.

Spermatozoan: A spermatozoan is a mature male gamete that develops in the seminiferous tubules of the testes, consisting of a head, a midpiece, and a tail.

Ejaculatory duct: This is the passage formed by the junction of the duct of the seminal vesicles and the vas deferens through which semen enters the urethra.

Seminal vesicle: The seminal vesicle is one of a pair of saclike accessory glands located posterior to the urinary bladder in the male that provide nourishment for sperm.

Prostate: The prostate is a gland located below the neck of the bladder in males that surrounds the proximal portion of the urethra. It is a firm structure composed of muscular and glandular tissue. Its function is to secrete and store a clear fluid that makes up one-third of the volume of semen.

Testosterone: This is the hormone that causes males to develop the classic characteristics of axillary and pubic hair, deeper voice, and sperm production.

The Female Reproductive System

Ovary: The female gonad, called the ovary, is located in the pelvis in which the ova, or germ cells, are formed. There are two ovaries, each covered with a single layer of epithelium. The ovarian follicle wall secretes estrogen.

Ovum: This is a mature female gamete.

Ovulation: This is the expulsion and release of a mature ovum from a follicle in the ovary as a result of cyclic ovarian and pituitary endocrine function. Ovulation usually occurs about two weeks before the menstrual period.

Progesterone: This hormone maintains the uterine endometrium in the richly vascular state necessary for implantation and pregnancy.

Estrogen: This hormone initiates and maintains growth of the functional layer of the endometrium (the innermost layer of the uterus).

Menstrual cycle: The recurring twenty-eight-day cycle of change in the endometrium during which the decidual layer of the endometrium is shed, regrows, and proliferates.

Menopause: Menopause is the cessation of the reproduction cycle. Menstrual cycles stop naturally with the decline of cyclic hormonal production between the ages of thirty-five and sixty.

Gestation: This is the period of development of the fetus from the time of fertilization to birth.

*Some of the following questions are not directly addressed in this chapter, but are meant to act as a general review of subjects studied in various school curriculums.

Questions

NCETM (14%) NCETMB (16%)

General Knowledge of Body Systems

1. What is the deadliest type of skin cancer?
   A. squamous cell
   B. melanoma
   C. basal cell
   D. stratified cell

2. How many bones are in the body?
   A. 150
   B. 178
   C. 206
   D. 216

3. What part of the nail should be kept trim and cut for massage therapists?
   A. the lunula
   B. the free edge
   C. the epidermis
   D. nail bed

4. The skeletal system that is made up of the skull, ribs, and vertebrae is called the
   A. appendicular.
   B. osteopendicular.
   C. central.
   D. axial.

5. The oily substance that prevents the skin from drying out is called
   A. sebum.
   B. sudiforous.
   C. citrona.
   D. ceruminous.

6. The three pigments that help determine skin color are
   A. iron, melanin, and carotene.
   B. hemoglobin, lunula, and carotene.
   C. hemoglobin, melanin, and carotene.
   D. iron, hemoglobin, and carotene.

7. The largest organ of the body is the
   A. skin.
   B. lungs.
   C. liver.
   D. stomach.

8. The spongy part of the bone is called the
   A. compact bone.
   B. matrix.
   C. cancellous.
   D. osteoblast.

9. The powerhouse of a cell is the
   A. ribosomes.
   B. microtubules.
   C. lysosomes.
   D. mitochondria.

10. The mechanism of how a muscle contracts is called the
    A. Sliding Filament Theory.
    B. Cross Bridge Theory.
    C. glycolysis.
    D. Krebs Cycle.

11. Functions of our skeletal system include all of the following except
    A. support.
    B. storage of vitamins.
    C. blood cell formation.
    D. movement.

12. The lubricant for our joints is called
    A. serous fluid.
    B. cutaneous fluid.
    C. synovial fluid.
    D. mucosal fluid.

13. The medical name for the heart muscle is
    A. pericardium.
    B. myocardium.
    C. plexicardium.
    D. pleural cardium.

14. The neuron that carries impulses from skin to the brain are the
    A. sensory.
    B. motor.
    C. cranial.
    D. cervical.

15. In order for an activity to qualify as a reflex it must be all of the following EXCEPT:
    A. voluntary.
    B. purposeful.
    C. stereotyped.
    D. predictable.

16. When blood leaves the heart it goes through the following vessels in order:
    A. arterioles, venules, capillaries, veins, arteries
    B. arteries, arterioles, capillaries, venules, veins
    C. arteries, capillaries, venules, veins, arterioles
    D. arterioles, arteries, capillaries, veins

17. The number of cervical nerves is
    A. seven.
    B. eight.
    C. twelve.
    D. five.

18. The part of the brain that serves as the cardiac and respiratory centers is the
    A. medulla oblongata.
    B. pons.
    C. midbrain.
    D. hypothalamus.

19. The top two chambers of the heart are called
    A. ventricles.
    B. vesicles.
    C. arteries.
    D. atria.

20. Once the blood exits the right ventricle, it goes to the
    A. lungs.
    B. aorta.
    C. right atrium.
    D. muscles of the body.

21. The deoxygenated blood from the body enters what part of the heart first?
    A. the left atrium
    B. the left ventricle
    C. the right atrium
    D. the right ventricle

22. The vessel that takes blood from the heart to the lungs is called the
    A. pulmonary vein.
    B. pulmonary artery.
    C. capillaries.
    D. None of the above are correct.

23. The large vessel that takes blood from the heart to the rest of the body is the
    A. coronary vessels.
    B. aorta.
    C. vein.
    D. pulmonary vein.

24. The central nervous system is made up of
    A. the nerves of the limbs.
    B. the ganglia and the spine.
    C. sensory nerves.
    D. brain and spinal cord.

25. The top number in the blood pressure is
    A. when the heart is contracted.
    B. the diastolic.
    C. the systolic.
    D. Both A and C are correct.
    E. Both A and B are correct.

26. The _____ system helps to slow heart rate, lower blood pressure, and slow down the functions of the body.
    A. sympathetic
    B. parasympathetic
    C. central
    D. peripheral

27. The _____ glands have ducts.
    A. endocrine
    B. endocephalitis
    C. exocrine
    D. exoscopic

28. _____ refers to the sum of all the chemical reactions occurring in the body.
    A. Homeostasis
    B. Metabolism
    C. Negative feedback
    D. Catabolism

29. The connective tissue that covers the bone is called
    A. fascia.
    B. pericardium.
    C. periosteum.
    D. fibrosteum.

30. The long shaft of a bone is called the
    A. diaphysis.
    B. epiphysis.
    C. osteocytes.
    D. osteophysis.

31. Another name for cerebrovascular accident is
    A. heart attack.
    B. blockage.
    C. stroke.
    D. None of the above are correct.

32. A clot traveling through a blood vessel is called a/an
    A. thrombus.
    B. embolus.
    C. infarction.
    D. phlebitis.

33. How many pairs of cranial nerves do we have?
    A. twelve
    B. thirty-one
    C. six
    D. thirty-two

34. The sutures in the skull are types of
    A. fibrous joints.
    B. diarthrosis joints.
    C. cartilaginous joints.
    D. synovial joints.

35. What is the proper order for a reflex arc?
    A. sensory organ, efferent neuron, interneuron, afferent neuron, effector
    B. sensory organ, efferent neuron, afferent neuron, interneuron, effector
    C. sensory organ, afferent neuron, interneuron, efferent neuron, effector
    D. afferent neuron, sensory organ, interneuron, effector organ, efferent

36. Which nerve roots make up the sciatic nerve?
    A. L2–L4
    B. S1–S4
    C. L4–S3
    D. L2–L5

37. What is known as the pacemaker of the heart?
    A. Purkinje fibers
    B. sino-atrial node
    C. atrioventricular node
    D. mitral node

38. The longest portion/structure of the digestion system is
    A. stomach.
    B. large intestine.
    C. small intestine.
    D. esophagus.

39. The medulla oblongata in the brainstem contains which of the following centers
    A. cardiac.
    B. motor.
    C. special senses.
    D. vision.

40. Bile produced in the liver helps with
    A. breaking down proteins.
    B. creating fats.
    C. breaking down fats.
    D. creating glucose.

41. An example of a sesmoid bone is the
    A. vertebra.
    B. ischium.
    C. patella.
    D. navicular.

42. The ileocecal valve is located
    A. between the small and large intestines.
    B. between the stomach and the duodenum.
    C. at the distal end of the esophagus.
    D. between the colon and the rectum.

43. When in "fight or flight" mode, which system is activated?
    A. sympathetic nervous system
    B. central nervous system
    C. parasympathetic nervous system
    D. peripheral nervous system

44. In which cavity are the lungs located?
    A. dorsal
    B. thoracic
    C. abdominopelvic
    D. respiratory

45. Oxygen attaches to _____ in order to be transported in the blood stream.
    A. iron
    B. tyrosine
    C. hemoglobin
    D. erythrocytes

46. Body temperature is regulated in which area of the brain?
    A. midbrain
    B. thalamus
    C. medulla oblongata
    D. hypothalamus

47. Which of the following is the breaking down phase of metabolism?
    A. anabolism
    B. homeostasis
    C. catabolism
    D. mastication

48. Which gland is on top of the kidneys?
    A. thyroid
    B. adrenal
    C. pancreas
    D. gall bladder

49. The "powerhouse" of the cell is called the
    A. mitochondria.
    B. myofilaments.
    C. myofibrils.
    D. myocytes.

50. The serous membranes
    A. line the inside of blood vessels.
    B. are found inside the heart muscle.
    C. cover the myelin sheath.
    D. surround the internal organs.

51. The diaphysis of long bones is mostly made up of
    A. cancellous bone.
    B. spongy bone.
    C. compact bone.
    D. medullary.

52. When bones grow, most of the growth takes place at the
    A. epiphysial plates.
    B. diaphysis plates.
    C. compact bone.
    D. osteocytes plate.

53. The cranial nerve responsible for carrying impulses to the face is the
    A. vagus.
    B. valgus.
    C. trigeminal.
    D. abducens.

54. When the heart is contracted, this correlates to which number in the blood pressure?
    A. the diastolic
    B. the systolic
    C. the bottom number
    D. Both A and C are correct.

55. Which hormone is activated in fight or flight?
    A. acetylcholine
    B. epinephrine
    C. adrenocorticotropic hormone
    D. estrogen

56. Which of the following is not a function of the integumentary system?
    A. protection
    B. storage of minerals
    C. thermal regulation
    D. excretion

57. Urine passes from the kidney to the bladder via the
    A. ureter.
    B. urethra.
    C. urinal canal.
    D. nephron.

58. The central nervous system is made up of
    A. twelve cranial nerves.
    B. nerves to the arms and legs.
    C. spinal cord and brain.
    D. spinal cord and motor nerves.

59. The pyloric sphincter is located
    A. at the end of the large intestines.
    B. at the sigmoid.
    C. between the stomach and the duodenum.
    D. between the esophagus and the stomach.

60. The amount of air moved into or out of the lungs during relaxed breathing is called the
    A. tidal volume.
    B. residual volume.
    C. vital capacity.
    D. total lung capacity.

61. Urine that is a dark gold color is sometimes due to
    A. too little vitamin B.
    B. too much vitamin A.
    C. too much vitamin B.
    D. None of the above are correct.

62. The exchange of gases between the blood supply and the body cells is called
    A. external respiration.
    B. ventilation.
    C. tapotement.
    D. internal respiration.

63. Each lung has one tube that branches off from the trachea. These tubes are called the
    A. bronchiole tubes.
    B. trachea.
    C. bronchial tubes.
    D. C-rings.

64. The lung that is shorter and wider is the _____ lung, and the lung that has two lobes is the _____ lung.
    A. left; right
    B. right; left
    C. left; left
    D. right; right

65. Urine is mostly made up of
    A. water.
    B. urea.
    C. ammonia.
    D. None of the above are correct.

66. Inflammation of the kidneys is called
    A. renal disease.
    B. nephritis.
    C. glomerularitis.
    D. uritis.

67. Another term for throat is
    A. larynx.
    B. trachea.
    C. esophagus.
    D. pharynx.

68. Which of the following is NOT a reason for needing sinuses in the skull
    A. to give resonance to the voice.
    B. to humidify and maintain the temperature of the air.

C. to vary the pitch of the voice.
D. to lighten the bone structure of the head.

69. The area where most digestion takes place is the
    A. large intestine.
    B. pylori.
    C. fundus.
    D. small intestine.

70. The only organ that can regenerate and continue to function if up to seventy-five percent is lost either due to surgery or disease is the
    A. colon.
    B. pancreas.
    C. liver.
    D. stomach.

71. The rhythmic contraction of the muscles in the alimentary canal that helps push the food through the digestive system is called
    A. peristalsis.
    B. vomiting.
    C. digestion.
    D. colitis.

72. When the veins around the anus or lower rectum are swollen and inflamed, it is called
    A. fistulae.
    B. hemorrhoids.
    C. pruritus ani.
    D. None of the above are correct.

73. The most basic level of structural organization of the body is
    A. chemical.
    B. cellular.
    C. tissue.
    D. epithelial.

74. The thyroid, parathyroid, and pancreas are organs of which system?
    A. digestive
    B. lymphatic
    C. endocrine
    D. exocrine

75. The relationship between physiology and anatomy is
    A. anatomy is the function and physiology is the structure.
    B. anatomy is the structure and physiology is the function.
    C. anatomy varies from person to person, while physiology is the same in all.
    D. physiology varies from person to person, while anatomy is the same in all.

76. The cuneiform and cuboid are both in which group?
    A. pelvis
    B. carpals
    C. metacarpals
    D. tarsals

77. Medullary canals are found in what type of bones?
    A. flat
    B. sesmoid
    C. short
    D. long

78. A police officer might overstress what endocrine function?
    A. pineal
    B. pancreas
    C. adrenals
    D. parasympathetic

79. Another name for the sac around the heart is
    A. periosteum.
    B. pleural fascia.
    C. myocardium.
    D. pericardium.

80. A motor neuron and all the muscle fibers that it innervates is called
    A. neuromuscular junction.
    B. neurotransmitter synapse.
    C. motor unit.
    D. reflex arc.

81. Aromatherapy stimulates the
    A. chemoreceptors.
    B. nocioceptors.
    C. proprioceptors.
    D. neuroreceptors.

82. The median nerve is a part of the
    A. sacral plexus.
    B. lumbar plexus.
    C. cervical plexus.
    D. brachial plexus.

83. When placing your hand on a hot stove, which nerve tells the brain that the stove is hot?
    A. motor nerve
    B. proprioceptive nerves
    C. sensory nerves
    D. chemoreceptors

84. Arteriosclerosis falls in the family of
    A. coronary artery disease.
    B. chronic obstructive pulmonary disease (COPD).
    C. scleroderma.
    D. pulmonary disease.

85. The lymphatic system's main ducts are called the
    A. aorta.
    B. thoracic.
    C. hepatic.
    D. nephron.

86. Lymph is more easily transported through the body in healthy people by
    A. movement.
    B. lymphatic drainage massage.
    C. cryotherapy.
    D. drinking more fluids with electrolytes.

87. Another name for the windpipe is the
    A. trachea.
    B. esophagus.
    C. sigmoid.
    D. cecum.

88. The gas exchange between the blood and the muscles is called
    A. internal respiration.
    B. external respiration.
    C. hemolysis.
    D. oxidation.

89. Oxytocin is secreted by the
    A. pituitary.
    B. ovaries.
    C. prostate.
    D. hypothalamus.

90. Androgens are secreted by the
    A. adrenals.
    B. gonads.
    C. thymus.
    D. Both A and B are correct.

91. What glands are also known as the sweat glands?
    A. apocrine glands
    B. holocrine glands
    C. ceruminous glands
    D. sebaceous glands

92. The filtering unit of the kidneys is called the
    A. ureter.
    B. urethra.
    C. nephron.
    D. pyramidalis.

93. The medial pectoral nerve innervates the
    A. teres minor.
    B. pectoralis major.

C. pectoralis minor.

D. Both B and C are correct.

94. The spleen usually lies at the level of ribs numbered
    A. nine to eleven.
    B. ten to twelve.
    C. three to five.
    D. five to seven.

95. What nerve innervates the diaphragm?
    A. phrenic
    B. vagus
    C. glossopharyngeal
    D. accessory

96. The skull sutures are what type of joint?
    A. synovial
    B. primary cartilaginous
    C. fibrous
    D. condylar

97. A myoma is
    A. a disease of the myelin sheath.
    B. a neurological disorder.
    C. a tumor in muscle tissue.
    D. a disease of the myocardium.

98. What is another name for a deadly malignant tumor of the epithelial tissue?
    A. basal cell
    B. melanoma
    C. myoma
    D. myalgia

99. Destruction of blood cells is called
    A. hemoglobin.
    B. hemorrhage.
    C. hyperacusis.
    D. hemolysis.

100. What ligament forms the false vocal cords?
    A. vestibular ligament
    B. arytenoid
    C. C-rings
    D. conus elasticus

101. What are the two major divisions of the autonomic nervous system?
    A. CNS and PNS
    B. sympathetic and parasympathetic
    C. motor and sensory
    D. None of the above are correct.

102. When sympathetic activity is in affect in the lungs, what actions will take place?
    A. bronchodilation and vasodilation
    B. brochoconstriction and vasoconstriction
    C. bronchodialation and vasoconstriction
    D. bronchoconstriction and vasodilation

103. The valve that separates the left atrium from the left ventricle is called the
    A. mitral.
    B. tricuspid.
    C. semilunar.
    D. Purkinje.

104. Through what type of valve does blood pass on its way out of the ventricles?
    A. mitral
    B. tricuspid
    C. semilunar
    D. Purkinje

105. The meninge layer that is closest to the brain is the
    A. arachnoid.
    B. dura mater.
    C. subarachnoid.
    D. pia mater.

106. The name of the cartilage that forms the "Adam's apple" is called
    A. hyoid.
    B. thyroid.
    C. cricoid.
    D. digastric.

107. The great saphenous vein empties into what other vein?
    A. inferior vena cava
    B. jugular
    C. femoral
    D. superior vena cava

108. Which kidney is positioned higher than the other?
    A. the right
    B. the left
    C. neither
    D. both

109. The three parts of the sternum include all of the following except
    A. body.
    B. manubrium.
    C. coracoid process.
    D. xiphoid process.

110. What is the name of the endocrine glands that lie posterior to the thyroid gland?
    A. adrenals
    B. parathyroid
    C. pancreas
    D. thymus

111. As the sciatic nerve moves distally, it becomes the
    A. lateral peroneal.
    B. medial peroneal.
    C. anterior peroneal.
    D. common peroneal tibia.

112. What organ lies in the upper left quadrant of the abdomen?
    A. liver
    B. appendix
    C. spleen
    D. gallbladder

113. How many pairs of sacral nerves do we have?
    A. one
    B. eight
    C. five
    D. twelve

114. The following are parts of a rib except
    A. body.
    B. neck.
    C. head.
    D. tubercle.
    E. All are parts of a rib.

115. What receives motor innervation from the hypoglossal nerve?
    A. eyes
    B. ears
    C. nose
    D. tongue

116. Another name for the mitral valve is the
    A. bicuspid.
    B. tricuspid.
    C. pulmonary semilunar.
    D. aortic semilunar.

117. Warts are
    A. a contagious infection of the epidermal layer of skin.
    B. a noncontagious infection of the subcutaneous layer of the skin.
    C. a noncontagious infection of the epidermal layer of the skin.
    D. a contagious infection of the subcutaneous layer of the skin.

118. What hormone is produced by the pineal gland?
    A. melatonin
    B. melanin
    C. prolactin
    D. insulin

119. A birthmark or mole is a
    A. vesicle.
    B. papule.
    C. nevus.
    D. papillae.

120. Cells that support and protect the neurons of the central nervous system are called
    A. dendrites.
    B. neuroglia.
    C. pia mater.
    D. dura mater.

121. Which of the following is NOT a function of the kidneys?
    A. produce cholesterol
    B. excretion of waste products in the urine
    C. maintain acid–base balance
    D. maintain water balance

122. Which pigment is found in the epidermis?
    A. melanin
    B. keratin
    C. iron
    D. myelin

123. The motor cortex of the brain is located in which lobe?
    A. occipital
    B. parietal
    C. temporal
    D. frontal

124. The largest organ in the body by weight is the
    A. liver.
    B. brain.
    C. skin.
    D. heart.

125. The control center of the cell that directs nearly all metabolic activities is the
    A. ribosome.
    B. endoplasmic reticulum.
    C. nucleus.
    D. mitochondrion.

126. The weight-bearing part of the vertebrae to which the disk attaches is called the
    A. centrum.
    B. body.

C. lamina.

D. Both A and B are correct.

127. Which of the following will not affect the para-sympathetic nervous system?
A. increased gastrointestinal motility
B. decreased heart rate
C. increased respiratory rate
D. decreased blood pressure

128. Blood cells are formed by a process called
A. hemocytopoiesis.
B. hemobirthocytosis.
C. hemocytogenesis.
D. Both A and C are correct.

129. The most numerous blood cells with the function of transporting oxygen and a small amount of carbon dioxide in the blood are called
A. hemoglobin.
B. erythrocytes.
C. thrombocytes.
D. leukocytes.

130. When a pathogen is absorbed rather than "eaten" by cells, the process is known as
A. pinocytosis.
B. phagocytosis.
C. fibrinogen.
D. exocytosis.

131. Which of the following are mechanisms for blood clotting?
A. platelet plug
B. coagulation
C. vascular spasm
D. All of the above are correct.

132. The "universal donor" is which type of ABO blood group?
A. A
B. B
C. AB
D. O

133. The valves located between both ventricles and their adjacent arteries are called the
A. tricuspid valves.
B. mitral valves.
C. sinoatrial valves.
D. semilunar valves.

134. The main part of the heart's conducting system is the
A. SA node.
B. AV bundle.
C. AV node.
D. All of the above are correct.

135. The majority of heart rate changes are controlled by the cardiac center located where?
A. the SA node
B. the medulla oblongata
C. the AV node
D. the Perkinje bundle

136. When the diameter of the vascular lumen enlarges, it is called
A. vasoconstriction.
B. vasodialation.
C. myocardial infarction.
D. endocardial fibrosis.

137. The expansion effect that occurs in the arteries when blood is pushed forward due to contraction of the left ventricle is called
A. cardiac cycle.
B. fibrillation.
C. tachycardia.
D. pulse.

138. The pressure exerted by blood on an arterial wall during the heart contraction phase is called
A. vascular pressure.
B. blood pressure.
C. arterial pressure.
D. All of the above are correct.

139. In which artery is blood pressure the most frequently taken?
A. brachial
B. carotid
C. radial
D. femoral

Answers and Explanations

General Knowledge of Body Systems

NCET M (14%) NCETMB (16%)

1. **B** Melanoma can get deep into the skin through many layers and invade body systems and organs.

2. **C** There are 206 bones in the human body: 80 in our axial skeleton and 126 in the appendicular skeleton.

3. **B** The lunula is the half moon whitish area at the base of the nail, the nail bed is the part attached to the finger, and the epidermis is

a layer of skin, so the free edge is the part that extends over the finger and needs to be trimmed by massage therapists.

4. **D** Osteopendicular is not a word. Central is usually used when discussing the central nervous system. The appendicular system is made up of the bones of the extremities.

5. **A** Sudiforous is related to the sweat glands, ceruminous is the ear wax, and citrona is not a word.

6. **C** Iron doesn't give color, hemoglobin does. Carotene gives the yellowish/orange tint, and melanin helps determine the darkness of the skin. Lunula is a part of the finger nail.

7. **A** The skin can take up surface area of twenty-two square feet and weighs about nine pounds.

8. **C** Compact bone is the hard surface of the bone, matrix is the gelatinous material inside cells, and osteoblasts are a cell that help to build bone.

9. **D** The ribosomes hold half of the DNA, the microtubules are the "skeleton" of the cell, and the lysosomes break down particles.

10. **A** The Sliding Filament Theory explains how, with enough ATP, the myosin attaches to the actin and pulls the actin towards the middle, thus "sliding" the actin over each other. Glycolysis is looking at cellular aerobic versus anaerobic activity, and the Kreb's Cycle describes how ATP is formed.

11. **B** The skeletal system stores minerals such as calcium—not vitamins.

12. **C** Serous fluid is lubricant around our organs.

13. **B** Pericardium is the sac around the heart. The other words are made up. Remember, "myo" means muscle, and "cardio" means heart. Together they equal heart muscle.

14. **A** Motor nerves tell the muscle or organ what to do. The brain sends the message to the organ or muscle via the motor nerve. The sensory nerve sends the message to the brain if something is hot, cold, hard, soft, etc.

15. **A** A reflex is not voluntary, it is involuntary. Think of blinking the eye—it just happens even when we try to stop it. It serves a purpose—lubrication of the eyes. It is sterotyped (it happens the same each time); and it is predictable (we know it will happen again and again).

16. **B** Arterioles are small arteries; venules are small veins. Where the two meet, they are called

capillaries, which is where the exchange of oxygen between the bloodstream and the tissue takes place.

17. **B** There are seven cervical vertebrae but eight cervical nerves.

18. **A** All are a part of the brainstem, but the medulla oblongata is the cardiac and respiratory center.

19. **D** Atriums are on top; ventricles are on the bottom.

20. **A** Blood goes to the lungs via the pulmonary artery ("a" in artery, "a" in away from the heart). Once in the lungs, oxygen is received. It then returns to the left atrium via the pulmonary vein, then the left ventricle, then the aorta, then out to the rest of the body.

21. **C** The deoxygenated blood (no oxygen, or venous blood) goes into the right atrium, then right ventricle, then the lungs via the pulmonary artery ("a" in artery, "a" in away from the heart). Once in the lungs, oxygen is received. It then returns to the left atrium via the pulmonary vein, then the left ventricle, then the aorta, and then out to the rest of the body.

22. **B** The deoxygenated blood (no oxygen, or venous blood) goes into the right atrium, then right ventricle, then the lungs via the pulmonary artery ("a" in artery, "a" in away from the heart). Once in the lungs, oxygen is received. It then returns to the left atrium via the pulmonary vein, then the left ventricle, then the aorta, then out to the rest of the body.

23. **B** The deoxygenated blood (no oxygen, or venous blood) goes into the right atrium, then right ventricle, then the lungs via the pulmonary artery ("a" in artery, "a" in away from the heart). Once in the lungs, oxygen is received. It then returns to the left atrium via the pulmonary vein, then the left ventricle, then the aorta, and then out to the rest of the body.

24. **D** The peripheral nervous system is made up of the limbs and extremities.

25. **D** The top number is the systolic and is when the heart is contracted. The bottom number is the diastolic and is when the heart is relaxed (which is why it is the lower of the two numbers).

26. **B** This system helps our bodies to slow down.

27. **C** The EX in exit and the EX in exocrine—the exocrine glands have an exit via the duct.

28. **B** This is a basic chemical/cellular physiology definition. Homeostasis is the balance of the

body and its functions. Catabolism is the breakdown of something, and negative feed-back is a psychology term for rewarding negative behavior.

29. **C** Fascia is the lining around muscles, blood vessels, and nerves that connects them to surround tissue to hold them in place; pericardium is the sac around the heart; fibrosteum is not a word.

30. **A** The epiphyses is the end of the long bone; osteocytes are bone cells, and osteophyses is a made-up term.

31. **C** A heart attack is also known as a myocardial infarction. A blockage may be a blood clot (thrombus) or buildup of plaque and could lead to a stroke or CVA if it lodges in the brain.

32. **B** A thrombus is a localized blood clot. An infarction is a heart attack, and phlebitis is inflammation of a vein.

33. **A** There are twelve pairs of cranial nerves and 31 pairs of spinal nerves.

34. **A** Diarthrosis joints are freely moveable joints and are also known as synovial joints. Cartilaginous joints are joints consisting of cartilage, such as the ear lobe or the tip of the nose.

35. **C** Sensory organ, afferent neuron, interneuron, efferent neuron, effector. For example, you place your hand on a hot stove. The nerves in the skin know it's too hot (sensory nerves), which sends a message towards the brain via the afferent neuron. The interneuron transmits what the brain wants done (to move the hand off the hot stove) to the efferent neuron which sends the information to the muscles that move the arm (effector), and the hand is removed from the stove.

36. **C** The sciatic nerve stems from L4–S3, which is why herniated discs in the lower back (lumbar vertebrae) often affect this nerve and cause pain down the posterior leg.

37. **B** The Purkinje fibers stimulate the ventricles to contract. The AV node helps to slow the rate to ensure the atrium has time to empty into the ventricles. There is a mitral valve, but not a mitral node.

38. **C** The stomach is a pouch; the large intestine is about five feet long; the small intestine is about twenty feet long; and the esophagus is about ten inches long.

39. **A** Cardiac. This is why punches to the back of the head/neck area can be fatal.

40. **C** Breaking down fats. This is why those who have had their gallbladder removed must eat a low fat diet or they might experience diarrhea.

41. **C** The vertebra is considered irregular, the ischium is also an irregular bone, and the navicular is considered a short bone.

42. **A** The sphincter between the stomach and the duodenum is the pyloric sphincter; the sphincter at the distal end of the esophagus is the cardiac sphincter.

43. **A** The central nervous system consists of the brain and spinal cord; the peripheral nervous system is the nerves to the extremities. The parasympathetic is the parachute that slows us down. The sympathetic is the system that speeds us up to prepare for fight or flight.

44. **B** The abdominopelvic is the ventral side of the body. There is no "respiratory" cavity. The dorsal cavity contains the brain and spinal cord.

45. **C** Iron is a mineral; tyrosine is a protein. Erythrocytes are red blood cells. Hemoglobin is the actual cell the oxygen binds to.

46. **D** The hypothalamus is the thermoregulatory center. The thalamus interprets pain and expresses it as rage or fear, and the midbrain sends impulses to the skeletal muscles that help us maintain tonus.

47. **C** Anabolism is the build-up phase of metabolism; homeostasis is maintaining a healthy balance; mastication is chewing.

48. **B** The thyroid is located in the throat area, the pancreas is just inferior to the stomach, and the gallbladder is in the left abdominal quadrant inferior to the liver.

49. **A** Cellular anatomy review. Myofilaments are the muscles of the cells. Myofibrils are the simplest unit of muscle cells.

50. **D** Serous membranes surround our internal organs so they do not "rub" against each other or create friction—which can be very painful.

51. **C** This provides strength in the bone. The epiphysis is mostly composed of cancellous bone (spongy bone).

52. **A** The only plates in bones are the epiphysial plates.

53. **C** There is no valgus nerve. The vagus affects the

abdominal organs and thoracic organs, and the abducens performs lateral eye movements.

54. **B** The top number is the systolic, and the bottom is the diastolic. The top number is when the heart is contracted, which is why it is the higher of the two numbers. The bottom number is when the heart is relaxed, which is why it is the lower of the two numbers.

55. **B** Adrenocorticotropic hormone regulates the adrenal cortex activity; epinephrine increases blood pressure by stimulating vasoconstriction that occurs during stress. By stimulating vasoconstriction instead of affecting cardiac output, it allows us the "energy" and ability to fight or flee.

56. **B** The integumentary system consists of the skin, hair, and nails. The skeletal system stores minerals.

57. **A** The urethra moves urine from the bladder to outside the body. Nephrons are the filters inside of the kidneys, and there is no such thing as a urinal canal.

58. **C** Twelve cranial nerves are only part of the CNS; nerves to the arms and legs and motor nerves are part of the peripheral nervous system.

59. **C** The cardiac sphincter is located between the esophagus and stomach.

60. **A** Residual volume is the amount of air left when you have exhaled all that you can (this volume prevents our lungs from collapsing). Vital capacity is the amount of air that can be forcibly inhaled and exhaled in one breath. Total lung capacity is the complete amount of air the lungs can hold.

61. **C** Too much vitamin B will be excreted via the urine and turn it a dark gold color; vitamin B is a water soluble vitamin. Dehydration will also turn urine a dark gold color but is not listed as a choice.

62. **D** External respiration is the exchange of gases from the air into the nose and mouth down to the lungs.

63. **C** The trachea is also known as the "airway," the bronchiole tubes branch off from the bronchi. The C-rings surround the trachea to provide support.

64. **B** The right lung is shorter due to the crowding of the liver. The left lung has two lobes while the right lung has three.

65. **A** Urine is made up of ninety-five percent water. The other five percent consists of various chemicals dissolved in water, the major one being urea.

66. **B** Renal disease is kidney disease/failure. This question is asking about inflammation, not failure.

67. **D** The esophagus is the tube that carries food to the stomach; the trachea is the airway; the larynx is the voice box.

68. **C** The vocal cords vary the pitch of the voice.

69. **D** The pylorus and fundus are both parts of the stomach.

70. **C** Think about all the living liver transplants!

71. **A** Vomiting is the opposite direction, digestion takes place once the food has gotten where it needs to go through the peristalsis, and colitis is inflammation of the colon.

72. **B** This is the basic definition of hemorrhoids.

73. **A** Chemical energy is ATP. Without chemical reactions, nothing else could take place, including the creation of a cell.

74. **C** The digestive system includes the stomach, esophagus, and small/large intestines; the lymphatic system includes the tonsils, thymus, lymph nodes, and spleen. Exocrine glands are sweat glands.

75. **B** This is a basic definition.

76. **D** The pelvis is the ischium, ilium, and pubis; the carpals are the trapezoid, trapezium, capitate, hamate pisiform, triquestrium, lunate, and scaphoid; the metacarpals are the five bones that make up the palm of the hand. The other tarsals include the talus, calcaneous, navicular and the third cuneiform.

77. **D** The medullary canal holds cells such as red blood cells and are found in the long bones.

78. **C** The adrenal glands help to kick in the "fight or flight" which many officers experience when dealing with a possible criminal situation.

79. **D** Periosteum is the fascia around bones, pleural fascia is part of the lungs, and myocardium is another name for the heart muscle.

80. **C** A reflex arc is the neural wiring of a reflex; a neuromuscular junction is the point where a motor neuron meets a skeletal muscle fiber.

81. **A** Chemoreceptors are those that are activated by chemical stimuli detecting smells, tastes, and chemistry changes in the blood.

82. **D** The median nerve runs down the arm from the brachial plexus.

83. **C** Sensory nerves "sense" pressure, texture, and temperature. The motor nerve is the impulse from the brain back to the hand to tell it to move.

84. **A** Arteriosclerosis is hardening of the arteries, which falls under coronary artery disease (CAD). COPD stands for chronic obstructive pulmonary disease (e.g., asthma, emphysema, chronic bronchitis); scleroderma is hardening of the skin and other epithelial tissues; and pulmonary disease is related to the lungs.

85. **B** The aorta is the largest artery in the body; the hepatic portal system is connected with the liver and gallbladder, and the nephron is the filter in the kidneys.

86. **A** Lymph is a very thick, milky fluid; movement is the best way to get it going in healthy and uninjured people.

87. **A** The esophogus is tube that carries food to the stomach; sigmoid and cecum are the colon.

88. **A** External respiration is the exchange of gases from the air into the nose and mouth down to the lungs.

89. **A** Oxytocin is secreted by the pituitary and stimulates smooth muscle contraction in the uterine wall and milk ejection from the mammary glands in females. In males, it stimulates contraction of the smooth muscle of the male reproductive tract.

90. **D** In the adrenal glands, gonadocorticoids release a small amount of androgens; gonadocorticoids are produced in the adrenal cortex.

91. **A** Apocrine glands are a type of sweat gland attached to hair follicles in the axilla and groin area. Ceruminous glands produce the waxlike material in the ears; sebaceous glands are oil glands. Holocrine glands are oil producing glands.

92. **C** Ureters come from the kidneys to the bladder; urethra goes from the bladder out the body.

93. **D** The axillary nerve innervates teres minor.

94. **A** The spleen is located in the left upper quadrant of the abdomen inferior to the diaphragm and adjacent to ribs nine through eleven.

95. **A** The other nerves listed are cranial nerves.

96. **C** Synovial joints are moveable joints, cartilaginous are cushions between bones or on the ends of moveable bones (hyaline), and condylar would be between the metacarpophalageal joints.

97. **C** Myo means muscle. Myocardium is the heart muscle; myelin sheath is around the nerves.

98. **B** Basal cell is the name of the cell that can become cancerous but generally isn't deadly. Myoma is a tumor of the muscle, and myalgia is another name for muscular pain.

99. **D** Hemoglobin is the red protein of red blood cells which binds to oxygen, hemorrhage is bleeding through a vessel, and hyperacusis is abnormal acuteness of hearing due to irritability of the sensory neural nerves.

100. **A** The arytenoid is cartilage of the larynx that rotates to allow for medial and lateral displacements of the vocal cords. The C-rings are in the trachea and offer its shape and protection. The conus elasticus is the elastic membrane that connects the vocal cords to the cricoid, thyroid, and arytenoid cartilage.

101. **B** The central nervous system and the peripheral nervous system are the two main parts of the overall nervous system. Motor and sensory nerves are two types of nerves of the system.

102. **C** Sympathetic activity is "fight or flight"; therefore, the body dilates the bronchiole tubes to allow more air in and constricts the blood vessels to funnel blood to the area most in need.

103. **A** The right ventricle is separated from the right atrium via the tricuspid valve. The semilunar valves are in the aorta and the pulmonary vessels. The Purkinje fibers are a bundle of branches of nerve fibers that conduct impulses to conduction fibers in the heart.

104. **C** Remember the semilunar valve is in the pulmonary vein (where the blood goes when leaving the right ventricle) and the aortic valve (where the blood leaves when leaving the left ventricle).

105. **D** Remember PAD—pia mater, arachnoid, dura mater—in that order from the closest to the brain to closest to the skull.

106. **B** The hyoid is a bone; cricoid lies inferior to the thyroid cartilage; and digastric is a muscle.

107. **C** This is a review of anatomy. The jugular is in the neck; the great saphenous is in the leg. First, it has to get to the femoral vein before in can go into the inferior vena cava and return to the heart.

108. **B** The right kidney is lower than the left because the liver takes up space on the right side.

109. **C** The coracoid process is part of the scapula.

110. **B** Adrenals are on the kidneys; pancreas is on the right side below the stomach; and the thymus is posterior to the sternum.

111. **D** As the common peroneal tibial nerve, the tibial component is formed from the anterior dividions of the sciatic nerve. The common fibular (peroneal) nerve is formed from the posterior division of the sciatic nerve.

112. **C** The other three are on the right side.

113. **C** We have eight cervical, twelve thoracic, five lumbar, five sacral, and one coccygeal.

114. **E** All of the parts listed are a part of the rib. The head attaches to the body of the vertebrae, the neck is between the head and the tubercle of the rib, the tubercle connects to the vertebral facet, and the body of the rib is the main portion of the rib.

115. **D** Cranial nerve XIII. Hypo means under, and glossal means tongue.

116. **A** This is because the two flaps of the valve resemble a mitre (the headpiece worn by bishops).

117. **A** The epidermis is the top layer of skin which is where warts are located. They are infectious and should be avoided during massage.

118. **A** Melanin is a pigment of the skin; insulin is produced by the pancreas; and prolactin is produced by the pituitary gland.

119. **C** A vesicle is a blister; a papule is a small, round, firm; elevated area in the skin, and a papillae is a projection such as on the tongue.

120. **B** Neuroglia wrap themselves around individual neurons forming a protective covering protecting both the central and peripheral nervous system. The pia mater and dura mater are meninges that protect the spinal cord. Dendrites are the "little trees" that direct impulses into the cell body.

121. **A** The liver helps with production of cholesterol.

122. **A** The other three choices are not pigments of the skin.

123. **D** The primary motor cortex is located in the frontal lobe of the brain along the precentral gyrus.

124. **C** The skin is the largest organ by square footage and by weight.

125. **C** The nucleus is the "brain" of the cell.

126. **B** There is no "centrum" of the vertebrae. The lamina is the portion between the transverse process and the spinal process.

127. **C** Remember the "para" in parachute—parachutes slow us down, so the parasympathetic system slows things down. Now if the gastrointestinal (GI) tract is slowed, it works efficiently, and food moves better to be excreted.

128. **D** Hemobirthocytosis is not a word.

129. **B** Hemoglobin is the red protein of red blood cells which binds to oxygen; thrombocytes are platelets that coagulate to stop bleeding; and leukocytes are white blood cells.

130. **A** Phagocytosis is the cell ingesting and digesting, exocytosis is the cell discharging particles too large to pass through diffusion, and fibrinogen helps to form the foundation of a clot.

131. **D** All are ways our bodies help to stop bleeding.

132. **D** AB is the universal recipient.

133. **D** The tricuspid valve is between the right atrium and right ventricle; the mitral valve is between the left atrium and the left ventricle. There is no sinoatrial valve although there is a sino-atrial node, or the SA node.

134. **D** All are important parts in the heart's conduction of impulses.

135. **B** Since the impulse needs to come from the brain, the answer is B. The other structures are located inside the heart or heart muscle.

136. **B** Vasoconstriction is when the lumen gets smaller; myocardial infarction is the medical term for a heart attack; and endocardial fibrosis is a disease of the heart.

137. **D** This is the pulse we feel in our neck or wrist. Tachycardia is a rapid heartbeat, and cardiac cycle is the contraction/relaxation cycle. Fibrillation is when the heart is beating so fast it cannot contract and it spasms.

138. **D** Blood pressure is a measurement of pressure on the walls of blood vessels. More specifically, when the heart is contracted, it is the systolic measurement of the blood vessel. Because it is measured within the arteries, it is also called arterial pressure. As arteries are blood vessels, it is also known as vascular pressure.

139. **A** The blood pressure cuff goes on the upper arm which would be brachial although the other locations listed have pulses.

Detailed Knowledge chapter 2
of Anatomy, Physiology, and Kinesiology

CHAPTER OUTLINE

Areas of Competence

Anatomical Position
Planes of Motion

Cavities of the Body

Body Movements
Types of Contractions
Muscle Movers

Biomechanics and Kinesiology
Muscles
Joints
Dermatomes

Nutrition
The Six Basic Nutrients

Questions

Answers and Explanations

- Muscle attachments
- Muscle fiber direction
- Tendons
- Fascia
- Joint structure
- Ligaments
- Bursae
- Dermatomes

B. Physiology

- Response of the body to stress
- Basic nutrition principles

C. Kinesiology

- Actions of individual muscles/muscle groups
- Types of muscle contractions (e.g., concentric, eccentric, isometric)
- Joint movements
- Movement patterns
- Proprioception

AREAS OF COMPETENCE

This chapter includes sections that correspond to the organization of the NCBTMB exam as follows:

NCTM (26%)

A. Anatomy
- Anatomical position and terminology (e.g., planes, directions)
- Individual muscles/muscle groups

NCTMB (26%)

Same as above with the following additions:
A. Anatomy

- Primary and extraordinary meridians
- Chakras

B. Physiology

- Meridians/channels (e.g., bladder, liver, spleen)

———
(See Chapter 7 for Eastern modalities.)

Strategies to Success

Study Skills

Find a good place to study!

Think about the atmosphere where you study best. Are you distracted by the slightest noise? Do you like a certain level of noise to keep you going and focused? Do you like studying alone or in groups? Also consider your comfort level. Do you find yourself drifting off when you study in bed or in a comfortable chair? Is studying at a desk too uncomfortable? There's no right place or way to study. Some people pace the halls while others find a secluded place where they won't be bothered. We do suggest finding a place that is well lighted. Eye strain can make you tired. Whatever place you pick, make sure it is right for you and study there regularly.

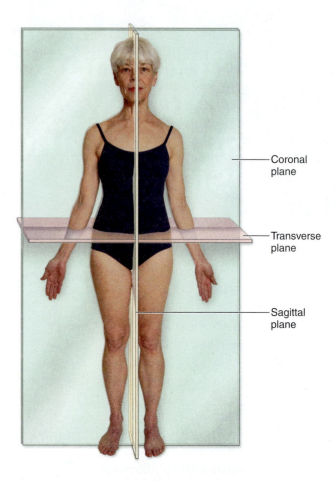

Figure 2-1 Anatomical position and planes of motion. *Source:* ©The McGraw-Hill Companies, Inc./Photo by JW Ramsey.

Anatomical Position

When learning and reviewing anatomical terms, remember to view the body from the anatomical position (Figure 2-1 and Table 2-1).

Planes of Motion

Imaginary sections or planes are made in the body in order to examine the internal anatomy and describe body position of one body part to another. These sections are called planes of motion. There are three planes of motion (see Figure 2-1).

Sagittal plane: This plane separates the body into left and right. Motions that occur in the sagittal plane run parallel to the plane (or an imaginary line splitting the body into left and right). Those motions would be flexion, extension, dorsiflexion, and plantar flexion.

TABLE 2-1

At a Glance: Anatomical Terms

Anatomical Position	Location
Superior (cephalad)	Higher than or above. Example: the heart is superior to the pelvis.
Inferior (caudal)	Lower than or below. Example: the patella is inferior to the pelvis.
Medial	Closest to the midline from anatomical position. Example: the adductor magnus is more medial than the iliotibial band.
Lateral	Farther from the midline from anatomical position. Example: the axillary border of the scapula is more lateral than the vertebral border of the scapula.
Proximal	Proximal and distal are dealing with the arms, hands, fingers, and feet. This is because when standing in the anatomical position, the arms are out at an angle. Therefore, they cannot be "superior" or "inferior." Proximal means closest to the midline or closer to the root of a limb. Example: the carpals are more proximal than the metacarpals.
Distal	Farther away from the midline in the arms, hands, fingers, feet or further from the root of a limb. Example: the phalanges of the foot are more distal than the metatarsals.
Anterior (ventral)	Closer to the front side of the body. Example: the pectoralis major is anterior to the trapezius.
Posterior (dorsal)	Closer to the back side of the body. Example: the erector spinae is posterior to the rectus abdominus.
Superficial	Closer to the skin surface. Also, if you think about a superficial cut, that is one that can be taken care of with a Band-Aid. Example: the trapezius is superficial to the rhomboids.
Deep	Closer to the core of the body. Again, think about a cut. If it is deep, it might require stitches. Example: the vastus intermedius is deep to the rectus femoris.

Transverse plane: This is the plane that separates the body into top and bottom. The motion that occurs in the transverse plane runs parallel to the plane (or an imaginary line splitting the body into top and bottom). This motion is rotation (medial, lateral, trunk).

Frontal plane: The frontal plane separates the body into front and back. Motions that occur in the frontal plane run parallel to the plane (or an imaginary line splitting the body into front and back). These motions are abduction, adduction, shoulder elevation, and shoulder depression.

Cavities of the Body

The body has two main cavities: the ventral and dorsal cavities (Figure 2-2).

Ventral cavity:
This cavity is more anteriorly located on the body and contains the following:

- The thoracic cavitiy (heart/lungs and area above the diaphragm)

- The abdominopelvic cavity (organs and structures below the diaphragm)

Dorsal cavity:
This cavity is more posterior on the body and contains the following:

- The cranial cavity (contains the brain)
- The spinal cavity (contains the spinal cord and vertebrae), also known as the vertebral canal.

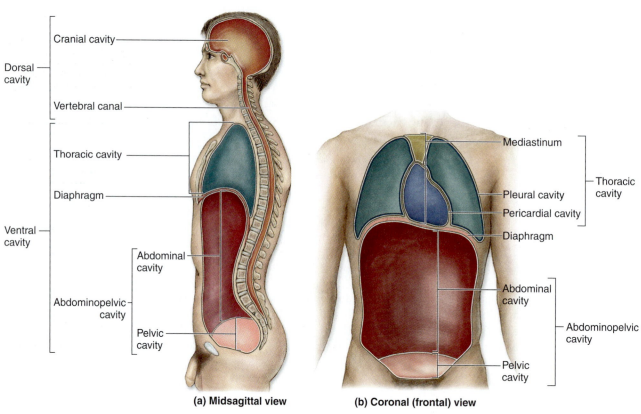

(a) Midsagittal view   **(b) Coronal (frontal) view**

Figure 2-2 The cavities of the body.

Body Movements

There are a variety of body movements. Remember, all body movements are from the anatomical position (Figures 2-3 A-D and Table 2-2). It is important as health care professionals that we understand each movement in order to be consistent with our clients.

TABLE 2-2

At a Glance: Body Movements and Their Descriptions

Movement	Description
Flexion	a decrease in the angle of a joint
Extension	an increase in the angle of a joint
Abduction	movement away from the midline
Adduction	movement towards the midline
Supination	turning the palms of the hands upward, or walking on the outer edge of the foot
Pronation	turning the palms of the hands downward, or walking on the inside edge of the foot
Medial rotation (internal rotation)	rotating towards the midline
Lateral rotation (external rotation)	rotating away from the midline
Elevation	raising the shoulders upward
Depression	lowering the shoulders
Dorsiflexion	pulling the toes upwards towards the lower leg (flatten the feet)
Plantar flexion	pointing the toes (remember the "P" in point; and the "P" in plantar flexion)
Eversion	soles of the feet away from the midline
Inversion	soles of the feet in towards the midline
Protraction	moving the scapula away from the spine, also called scapular abduction
Retraction	moving the scapula towards the spine, also called scapular adduction

Figure 2-3A

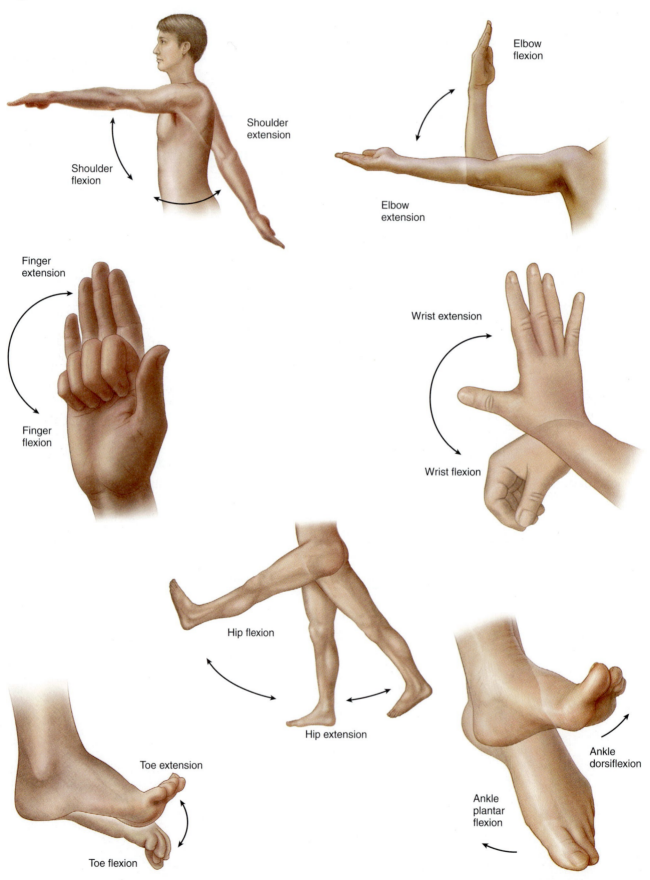

Figure 2-3B

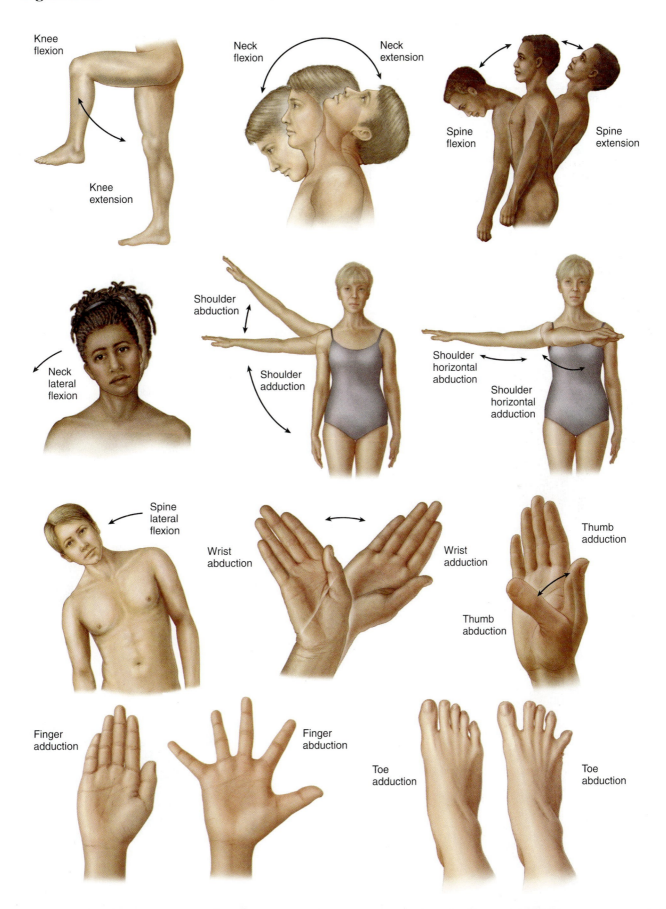

Figure 2-3C

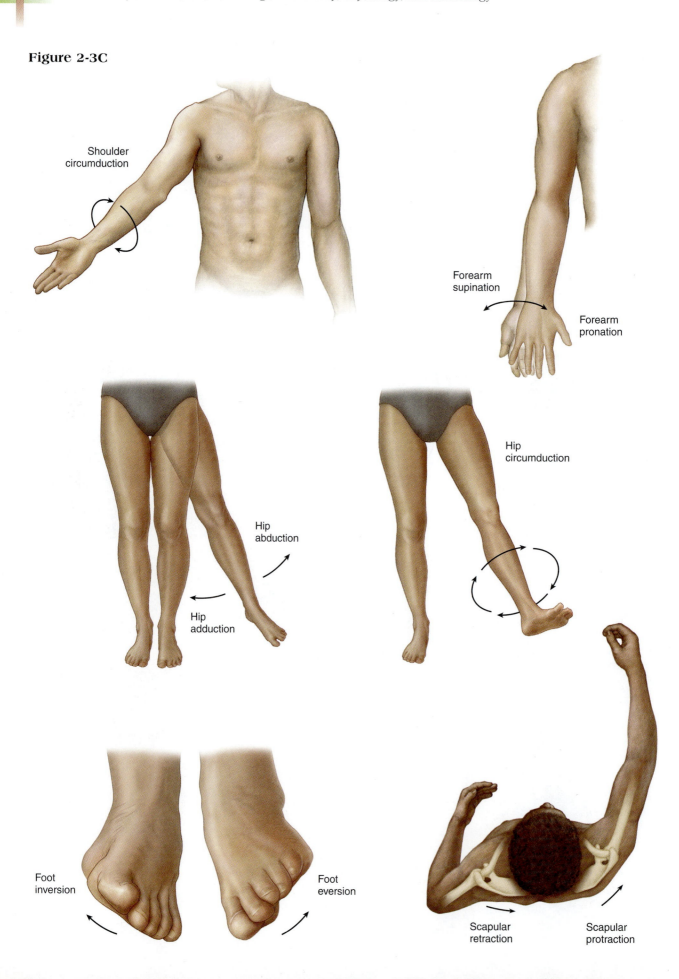

Figure 2-3D

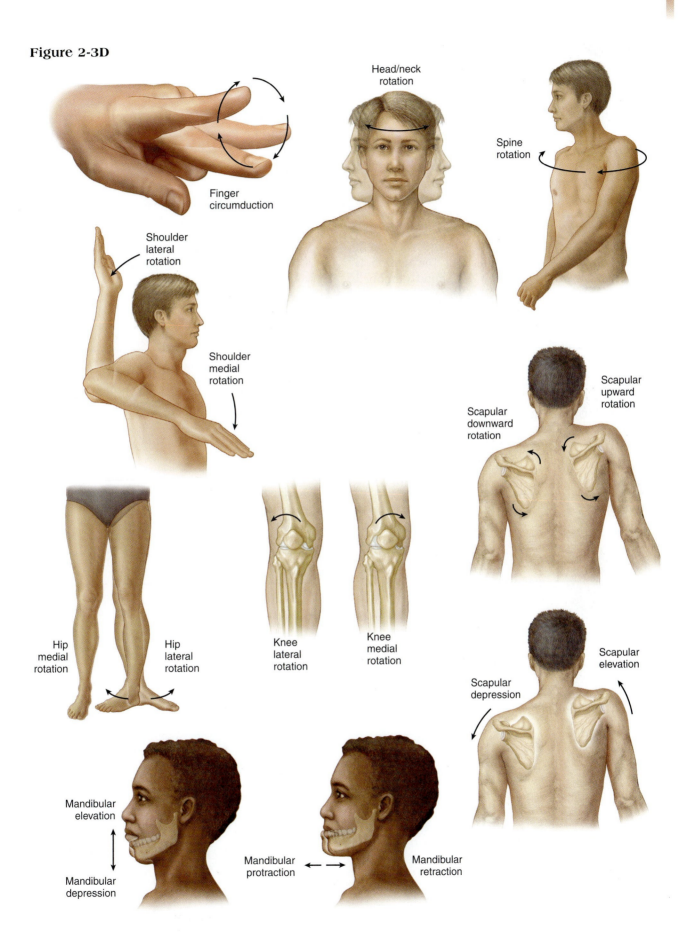

Finger circumduction

Head/neck rotation

Spine rotation

Shoulder lateral rotation

Shoulder medial rotation

Scapular downward rotation

Scapular upward rotation

Hip medial rotation

Hip lateral rotation

Knee lateral rotation

Knee medial rotation

Scapular depression

Scapular elevation

Mandibular elevation

Mandibular depression

Mandibular protraction

Mandibular retraction

Types of Contractions

A contraction is a shortening or tightening, as in a muscle (Table 2-3). The following list includes common contractions.

Isometric: (Iso = same; metric = length). This is when the muscle is contracting, but the joint/s is/are not moving. For example, push your hands together palm-to-palm. You feel the muscles contracting in your arms, but the shoulder, elbow, and wrist are not moving.

Isotonic: (Iso = same; Tonic = tension). Movement occurs with this type of contraction. The tension is either external force, such as a 50 pound dumbbell (the dumbbell "tension" will stay the same) or internal force (such as using weightlifting machines where the cam makes some movements easier than others). With internal force, the muscle tension stays the same throughout the range of motion. Internal force is generally seen in a gym setting. However, in our normal movements, we generally deal with external force, so that will be our focus. There are two types of isotonic contractions:

1. Eccentric—the lowering phase of movement. The muscles are contracting but lengthening, which allows us to put things down gently.

2. Concentric—the lifting phase of movement. The muscles shorten and contract.

TABLE 2-3

At a Glance: Muscle Contractions

Type of Contraction	Description
Isometric	Stabilizing—both agonist and antagonist exert the same amount of force preventing movement at the joint.
Isotonic	Movement at the joint occurs
1. concentric	1. The agonist (primary mover) shortens while contracting, otherwise known as the "up" phase
2. eccentric	2. The agonist (primary mover) is lengthening while still contracting, otherwise known as the "down" phase.

Muscle Movers

Agonists (primary movers): Agonists are the main muscle(s) doing the movements. These are usually the larger muscles since they have to be strong.

Assisters: The assister muscles help the primary movers in one of two ways:

1. Synergist—this helps the primary mover by moving the same way. If the primary mover is in a concentric contraction, so is the synergist. If the primary mover is in an eccentric contraction, so is the synergist.
2. Antagonist—this helps the primary mover by moving opposite. If the primary mover is in a concentric contraction, the antagonist is in an eccentric contraction.

Stabilizers: These muscles help prevent motion. We usually get hurt when our stabilizers become primary movers, such as in lifting something off the floor by bending at the waist instead of using our legs.

Connective tissue: The function of connective tissue is to support, protect, and connect other tissues. Types of connective tissue relating to the muscular system include tendons, ligaments, and cartilage.

Tendons: Tendons attach muscle to bone (for example, the Achilles tendon attaches the gastrocnemius to the calcaneous).

Ligaments: Ligaments attach bone to bone (for example, the anterior cruciate ligament attaches the femur to the tibia).

Cartilage: Cartilage provides the cushion between bones. An example is the two cartilages between the femur and the tibia of the knee.

See Figures 2-4 and 2-5 for diagrams of main muscles of the body. Remember, origins are the strong non-moveable ends of a muscle. Insertion is the moveable end. Generally, origins are closer to the center or midline of the body, and insertions are farther away from the midline.

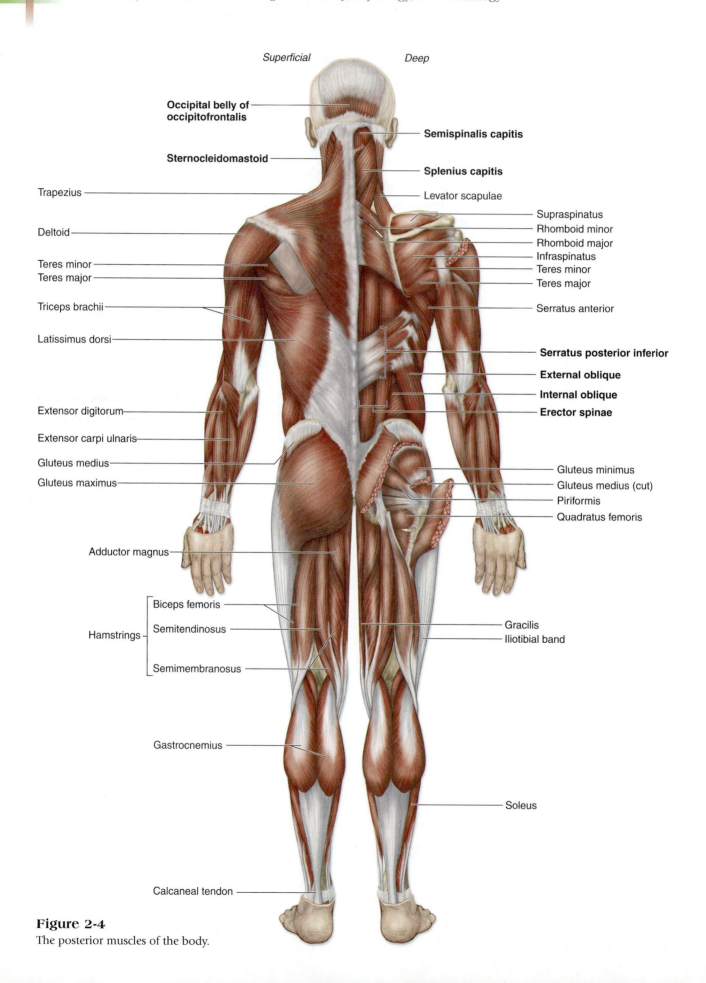

Figure 2-4

The posterior muscles of the body.

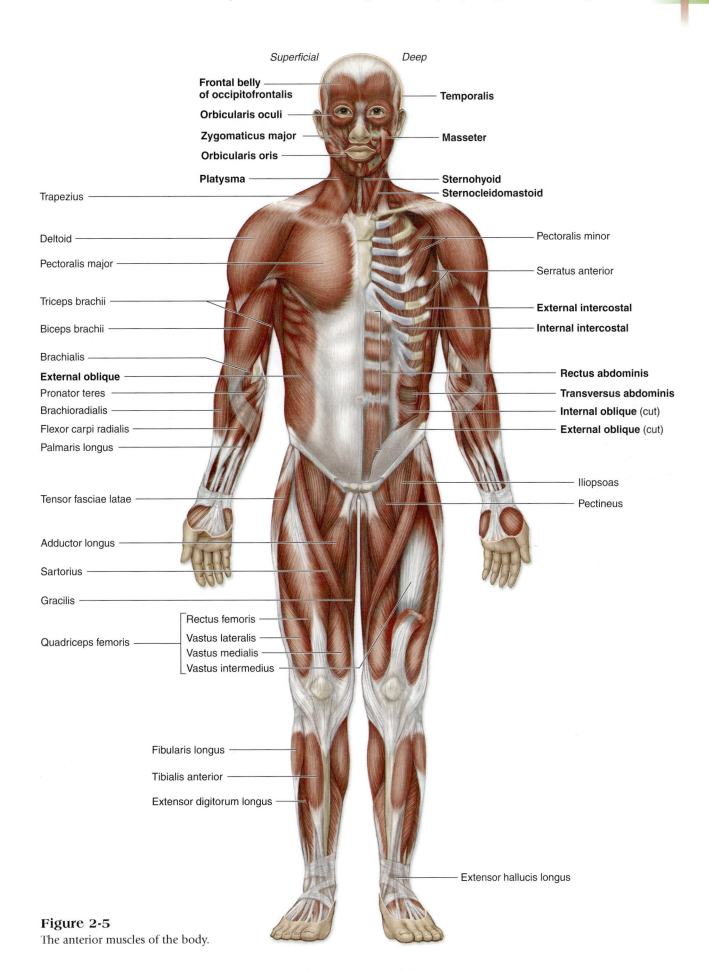

Figure 2-5
The anterior muscles of the body.

Biomechanics and Kinesiology

Biomechanics is the analysis of biological systems in mechanical terms, and kinesiology is the study of body movement. The body has muscle spindles and Golgi tendons to help us with body position (proprioception). The benefits of using proper body mechanics for massage include the following:

- Increased strength and power
- Increased pressure
- Decreased possibility of injury
- Enhanced quality and effectiveness of massage
- Increased career and life span as a therapist/bodyworker

Proprioception: Proprioception is the ability to know where your body is in space. For example, if you were to close your eyes and lift your leg up to hip level, you would know it was at hip level without having to look. See Chapter 1 for a detailed discussion.

Golgi tendons: Golgi tendons are nerve endings located within tendons near a muscle-tendon junction. They help keep us from over-contracting by sending signals to the inter-neurons in the spinal cord which in turn inhibit the actions of the motor neurons. This allows the muscle to relax, thus protecting the muscle and tendon from excessive tension damage. So if we try to lift an object that is too heavy, our muscles will respond so that we realize it is too heavy and drop it. Otherwise, we end up straining a muscle.

Muscle spindles: A muscle spindle is a stretch receptor found in the muscle which detects a stretching force in the muscle caused by a contraction. Muscle spindles help us by preventing muscles from over-stretching.

Muscles

Knowledge of muscle origins and insertions is a must for any massage therapist or bodyworker. Remember, origins are generally the stronger, non-moveable end of the muscle, while insertions are the weaker moveable end of the muscle. See Figure 2-6 and Table 2-4 for the main muscles of the face and head.

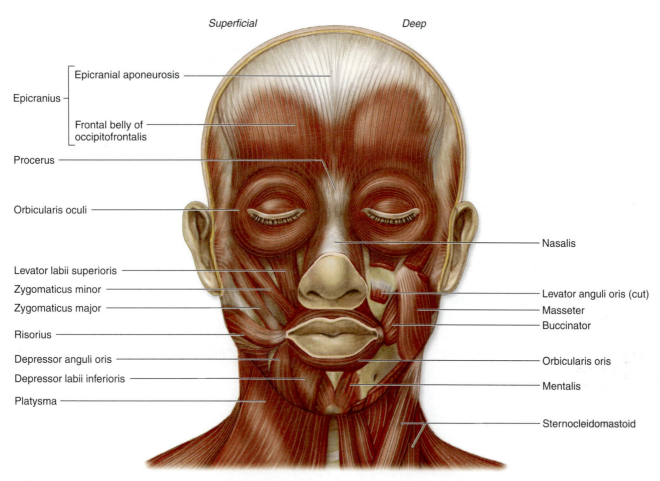

Figure 2-6 Muscles of facial expression and mastication.

TABLE 2-4

At a Glance: Muscles of the Face and Head

Muscle	Origin	Insertion	Action
Epicranius	Occipital bone	Skin and muscles around eye	Raises eyebrow
Orbiularis oculi	Maxillary and frontal bones	Skin around the eye	Closes eye
Orbicularis oris	Muscles near the mouth	Skin of lips	Closes and protrudes lips
Buccinator	Outer surface of maxilla and mandible	Orbicularis oris	Compresses cheeks inward
Zygomaticus	Zygomatic bone	Orbicularis oris	Raises corner of mouth
Platysma	Fascia in upper chest	Lower border of mandible	Draws angle of mouth downward
Masseter	Zygomatic arch	Angle and ramus of the mandible	Elevates the mandible
Temporalis	Temporal bone and lateral surface	Coronoid process of mandible	Closes jaw

Now, we will take a look at muscles that actually move the head (Figure 2-7). Notice that some of these muscles attach onto the spine, clavicle, and ribs to provide stabilization as well as movement at the neck and/or head. The name of the muscle often-times tells you the location. For example, splenius cervicus tells you there is an attachment on the cervical vertebrae (cervicus); splenius capitus tells you there is an attachment on the skull (capitus = head). See Table 2-5.

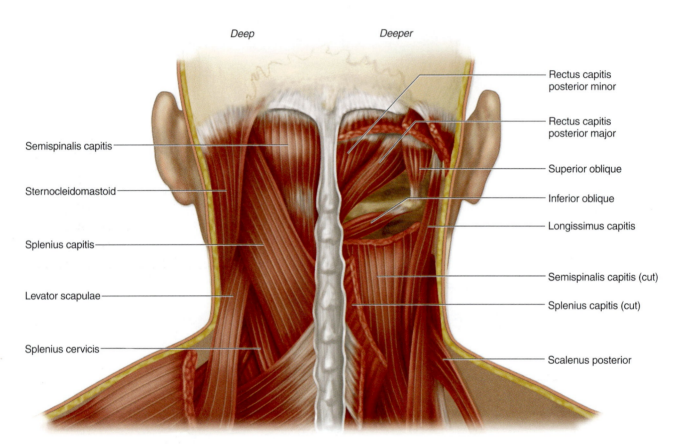

Figure 2-7 Posterior view of muscles that move the head.

TABLE 2-5

At a Glance: Muscles That Move the Head

Muscle	Origin	Insertion	Action
Sternocleidomastoid	Manubrium of sternum, medial one-third of clavicle	Mastoid process of temporal bone	Unilaterally: laterally flexes neck and rotates head to one side Bilaterally: flexes neck and assits in forced inspiration
Splenius capitis	Nuchal ligament, spinous process of C7–T3	Mastoid process, inferior nuchal line-lateral region	Unilaterally: rotates the head and laterally flexes the neck Bilaterally: extends the head
Splenius cervicus	Spinous processes of T3–T6	Transverse processes of C1–C3	Unilaterally: rotates the head and laterally flexes the neck Bilaterally: extends the head
Scalenes posterior	Tranverse processes of C5–C6	Rib 2 (superior	Unilaterally: laterally flexes
Scalenes anterior	Transverse process of C3–C6	Rib 1 (superior surface)	Unilaterally: laterally flexes the neck and rotates the head
Scalenes medius	Transverse process of C2–C7	Rib 1 (superior surface)	Unilaterally: laterally flexes the neck and rotates the head Bilaterally: elevates the first rib during inhalation

Remember, the shoulder girdle muscles either attach to or move the scapula, or they attach to the clavicle. Shoulder joint muscles only move the shoulder joint and have no action or attachment to the scapula or the clavicle (Table 2-6). See Figures 2-8 and 2-9 for muscles that move the pectoral girdle and the trunk.

TABLE 2-6

At a Glance: Muscles That Move the Pectoral Girdle and Trunk

Muscle	Origin	Insertion	Action
Trapezius	External occipital protuberance, superior nuchal lines, nuchal ligament, spinous processes of C7–T12	Lateral one-third of clavicle, acromion process, scapular spine	Upper fibers: extends the neck and head, elevates scapula, and upwardly rotates the scapula Bilaterally: extends the head and neck Middle fibers: retracts the scapula Lower fibers: depresses the scapula Unilaterally: laterally flexes the neck Bilaterally: rotates the head
Rhomboid major	Spinous processes of T2–T5	Vertebral border of scapula	Retracts the scapula and downwardly rotates the scapula
Rhomboid minor	Spinous processes of C7–T1	Vertebral border of the scapula	Retracts the scapula and downwardly rotates the scapula
Levator scapulae	Transverse processes of C1–4	Superior angle of the spine of scapula at the root	Unilaterally: elevates the scapula, downwardly rotates the scapula, laterally flexes the neck Bilaterally: extends head and neck
Serratus anterior	Ribs 1–8	Anterior medial border of the scapula	Protracts the scapula and upwardly rotates the scapula
Pectoralis minor	Ribs 3–5	Coracoid process of scapula	Depresses the scapula, protracts the scapula, downwardly rotates the scapula, and assists in forced inspiration
Internal oblique	Iliac crest, thoracolumbar fascia, inguinal ligament	Ribs 7–12, linea alba	Unilaterally: laterally flexes and rotates the vertebral column Bilaterally: flexes the vertebral column
External oblique	Ribs 5–12	Iliac crest, abdominal fascia, linea alba	Unilaterally: laterally flexes and rotates the vertebral column Bilaterally: flexes the vertebral column
Rectus abdominus	Pubic symphysis and pubic tubercle	Ribs 5–7 and xiphoid process	Flexes the vertebal column, compresses the abdominal contents
Transverse abdominus	Ribs 7–12, iliac crest, thoracolumnar aponeurosis, inguinal ligament	Abdominal aponeurosis, linea alba	Compresses the abdominal contents
Erector spinae	Spinous processes of C1–L5, nuchal ligament, posterior iliac crest, ribs 1–12, posterior sacrum	Mastoid process, ribs 1–12, transverse processes of C2–T8, occipital bone	Unilaterally: laterally flexes the vertebral column Bilaterally: extends the vertebral column and head
Quadratus lumborum	Posterior iliac crest	Ribs 12 (inferior surface), transverse process of L1–4	Unilaterally: laterally flexes the vertebral column and elevates the hip Bilaterally: extends the lumbar spine and anteriorly tilts the pelvis

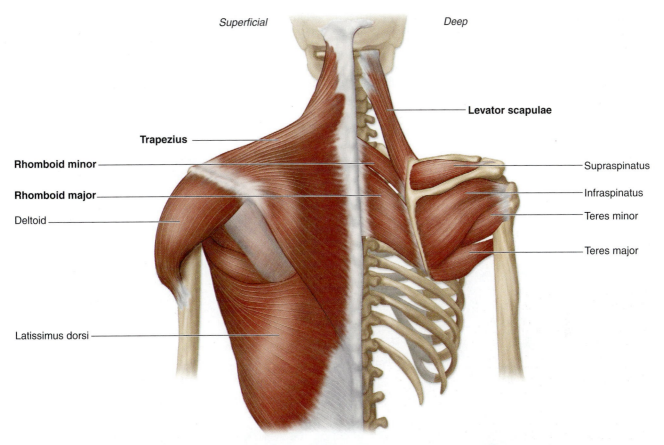

Superficial   *Deep*

Levator scapulae

Trapezius

Rhomboid minor   Supraspinatus

Rhomboid major   Infraspinatus

Deltoid   Teres minor

                                                       Teres major

Latissimus dorsi

Figure 2-8 Muscles of the posterior shoulder. The right trapezius is removed to show underlying muscles.

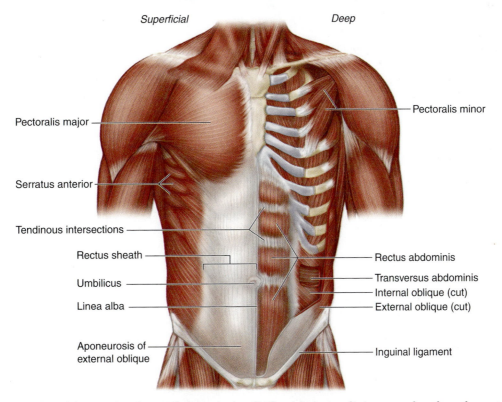

Superficial   *Deep*

Pectoralis major   Pectoralis minor

Serratus anterior

Tendinous intersections

Rectus sheath   Rectus abdominis

Umbilicus   Transversus abdominis
                                                       Internal oblique (cut)
Linea alba   External oblique (cut)

Aponeurosis of
external oblique   Inguinal ligament

Figure 2-9 Muscles of the anterior chest and abdominal wall. The right pectoralis is removed to show the pectoralis minor.

Figure 2-10 shows muscles that move the arm; however, notice that some of the muscles also affect the shoulder which would make them shoulder girdle muscles. Note that the rotator muscles are the SITS muscles and are listed in the order that they "sit" on the shoulder. The origin is the name of the fossa from which they originate. The insertion can be remembered by the subscapularis—it is "sub" standard and is the only rotator cuff muscle to attach to the lesser tubercle. The others are so great, they attach to the greater tubercle. See Table 2-7.

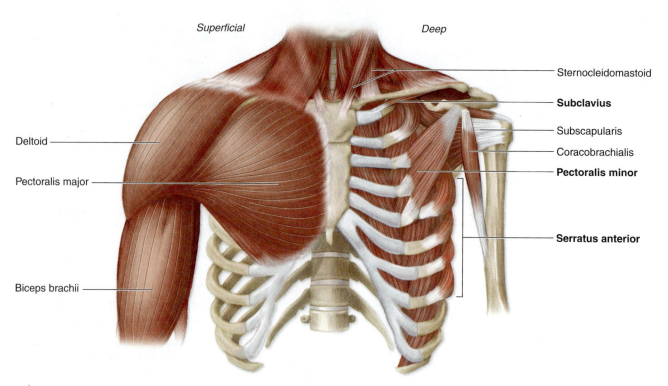

Superficial   *Deep*

Sternocleidomastoid

Subclavius

Subscapularis

Coracobrachialis

Pectoralis minor

Serratus anterior

Deltoid

Pectoralis major

Biceps brachii

Figure 2-10 Muscles of the anterior shoulder and arm.

TABLE 2-7

At a Glance: Muscles that Move the Arm

Muscle	Origin	Insertion	Action
Coracobrachialis	Coracoid process of the scapula	Medial humeral shaft	Flexes and adducts the shoulder
Pectoralis major	Medial half of clavicle edge of sternal body, ribs 1–8	Intertubercular groove of the humerus	Adducts the shoulder, medially rotates the shoulder, flexes the shoulder (clavicular fibers only), and extends the shoulder (sternal and costal fibers)
Teres major	Inferior half of the lateral border of the scapula	Intertubercular groove of the humerus	Teres major extends the shoulder, medially rotates the shoulder, adducts the shoulder
Latissimus dorsi	Spinous process of T6–L5, ribs 9–12, posterior iliac crest, and posterior sacrum	Intertubercular groove of the humerus	Extends the shoulder, medially rotates the shoulder, adducts the shoulder
Deltoid	Lateral third of clavicle, acromion process, scapular spine	Deltoid tuberosity of humerus	Anterior fibers: flex and medially rotate the shoulder Medial fibers: abducts the shoulder Posterior fibers: extend and laterally rotate the shoulder
Rotator Cuff Muscles			
Supraspinatus	Supraspinous fossa of the scapula	Greater tubercle of the humerus	Abducts the shoulder Stabilizes head of humerus in glenoid cavity
Subscapularis	Subscapular fossa of the scapula	Lesser tubercle of the humerus	Medially rotates the shoulder Stabilizes head of humerus in glenoid cavity
Infraspinatus	Infraspinous fossa of the scapula	Greater tubercle of the humerus	Laterally rotates the shoulder Adducts shoulder; extends shoulder, horizontally abducts shoulder
Teres minor	Superior half of the lateral border of the scapula	Greater tubercle of the humerus	Adducts the shoulder and laterally rotates the shoulder Extends shoulder; horizontally abducts shoulder; stabilizes head of humerus in glenoid cavity

Remember, many muscles' names tell you either the location (brachio = arm and radialis = radius bone), or how many origins they might have (bi = 2, so bicep has two origins), or the action (supinator supinates the forearm). See Figure 2-11a for muscles that move the anterior forearm (Table 2-8).

Generally speaking, the wrist/finger flexors are on the anterior side of the forearm, and the wrist/finger extensors are on the posterior forearm. See Figure 2-11b for muscles that move the posterior forearm (Table 2-8). Place your hand on the medial epicondyle, and you will feel muscles flexing when your flex

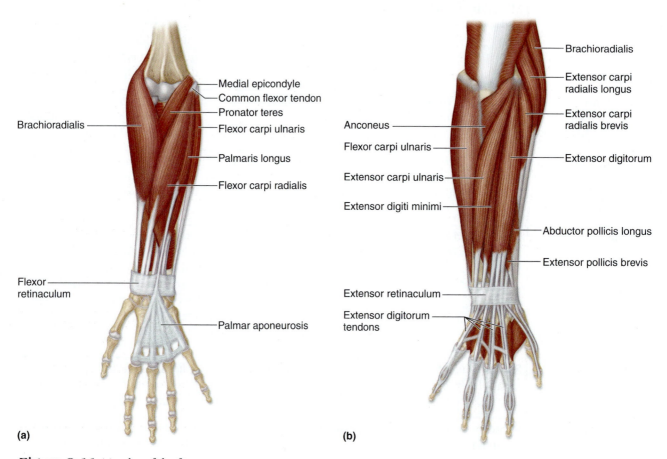

(a)

(b)

Figure 2-11 Muscles of the forearm.

TABLE 2-8

At a Glance: Muscles That Move the Forearm

Muscle	Origin	Insertion	Action
Biceps brachii	Long head: supraglenoid tubercle of scapula Short head: coracoid process of scapula	Radial tuberosity	Flexes the elbow, supinates the forearm, and flexes the shoulder
Brachialis	Distal anterior humeral shaft	Ulnar tuberosity	Flexes the elbow
Brachioradialis	Lateral supracondylar ridge of the humerus	Styloid process of radius	Flexes the elbow when the hand is in the neutral position
Triceps brachii	Long head: infraglenoid tubercle of the scapula Lateral head: posterior proximal humeral shaft Medial head: posterior distal humeral shaft	Olecranon process	Extends the elbow and extends the shoulder
Supinator	Lateral epicondyle of the humerus, proximal one-eighth of ulnar shaft, radial collateral ligament, and annular ligament	Proximal lateral radial shaft	Supinates the forearm
Pronator teres	Medial epicondyle of the humerus and the coronoid process of the ulna	Lateral proximal radial shaft	Pronates the forearm and flexes the elbow
Pronator quadratus	Anterior distal one-eighth of the ulnar shaft	Anterior distal one-eighth of the radial shaft	Pronates the forearm

your wrist. The medial epicondyle is the common origin for most wrist flexors. Now place your hand on the lateral epicondyle, and extend your wrist. The lateral epicondyle is the common origin for most wrist extensors. See Table 2-9 for muscles that move the wrist, hand, and fingers.

TABLE 2-9

At a Glance: Muscles That Move the Wrist, Hand, and Fingers

Muscle	Origin	Insertion	Action
Flexor carpi radialis	Lateral supracondylar ridge of the humerus	Bases of metacarpals 2–3	Flexes and abducts the wrist
Flexor carpi ulnaris	Medial epicondyle of the humerus	Base of metacarpal 5, pisaform, and hamate	Flexes and adducts the wrist
Palmaris longus	Medial epicondyle of humerus	Tranverse carpal ligament and palmar aponeurosis	Flexes the wrist and cups the palm
Flexor digitorum profundus	Anterior proximal three-fourths of the ulnar shaft	Distal phalanges of fingers 2–5	Flexes the fingers and the distal interphalangeal joint (DIP), the proximal interphalangeal joint (PIP), and the middle phalanx (MP) joints
Extensor carpi radialis longus and brevis	Longus: supracondylar ridge of the humerus	Longus: base of metacarpal 2	Extends and abducts the wrist
	Brevis: lateral epicondyle of the humerus	Brevis: base of metacarpal 3	distal interphalangeal joint proximal interphalangal joint middle phalanx
Extensor carpi ulnaris	Lateral epicondyle of the humerus	Base of metacarpal 5	Extends and adducts the wrist
Extensor digitoum	Lateral epicondyle of the humerus	Middle phalanges of the four fingers	Extends the wrist and extends the fingers at the DIP, PIP, and MP joints
Extensor pollicis longus and brevis	Longus: posterior ulnar shaft middle region, posterior radial shaft middle region, and interosseous membrane	Longus: distal phalanx of thumb	Extends the thumb
	Brevis: posterior radial shaft distal region and interosseous membrane	Brevis: proximal phalanx of thumb	
Flexor pollicis longus and brevis	Longus: anterior radial shaft middle region, interosseous membrane, and anterior ulnar shaft middle region	Longus: distal phalanx of thumb	Flexes the thumb
	Brevis: trapezium and transverse carpal ligament	Brevis: proximal phalanx of thumb	
Oppenens policis	Trapezium and transverse carpal ligament	Proximal phalanx of thumb	Flexes and adducts the thumb

Look for similarities among muscle groups. For example, the quadriceps group (rectus femoris, vastus medialis, vastus lateralis, and vastus intermedialis) all have a common insertion—the tibial tuberosity. See Table 2-10 for muscles that move the thigh and leg (Figures 2-12, 2-13, and 2-14).

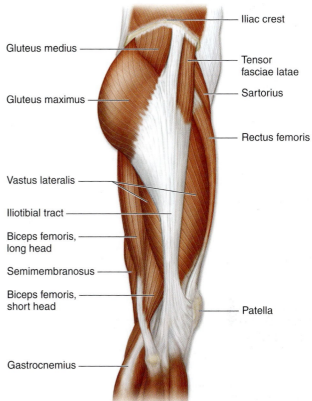

Figure 2-13 Muscles of the right lateral thigh.

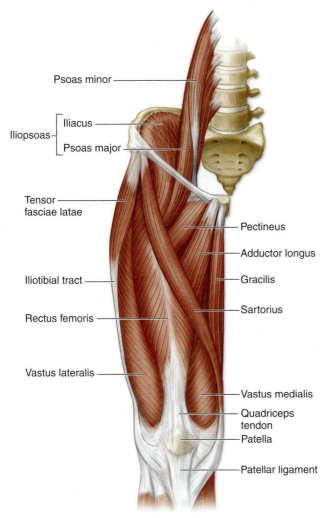

Figure 2-12 Muscles of the right anterior thigh.

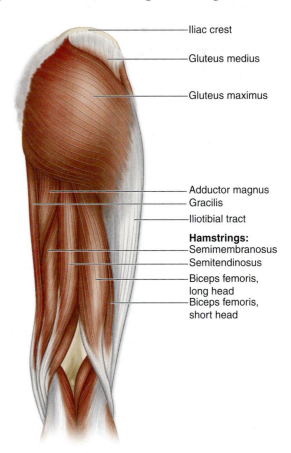

Figure 2-14 Muscles of the right posterior thigh.

TABLE 2-10

At a Glance: Muscles That Move the Thigh and Leg

Muscle	Origin	Insertion	Action
Psoas major	Transverse processes and vertebral bodies of T12–L5	Lesser trochanter	Unilaterally: laterally rotates the hip Bilaterally: flexes the hip and the vertebral column
Iliacus	Iliac fossa and anterior inferior iliac spine	Lesser trochanter	Flexes and laterally roates the hip Flexes hip; extends hip
Gluteus maximus	Posterior sacum, posterior coccyx, and posterior iliac crest	Glutal tuberosity (25%) and iliotibial band (75%)	Extends, laterally rotates, and abducts the hip
Gluteus medius	Superior gluteal line	Greater trochanter	Abducts and medially rotates the hip Flexes hip; extends hip
Gluteus minimus	Inferior gluteal line	Greater trochanter	Abducts and medially rotates the hip, and flexes hip
Tensor fasciae latae	Anterior iliac crest and anterior superior iliac spine	Iliotibial band	Abducts, flexes, and medially rotates the hip
Adductor longus	Pubic tubercle	Linea aspera	Adducts the hip, medially rotates hip
Adductor magnus	Ischial tuberosity, inferior pubic ramus, and ischial ramus	Linea aspera and adductor tubercle of the femur	Adducts, flexes, and extends the hip, and medially rotates hip
Adductor brevis	Inferior pubic ramus	Linea aspera	Adducts the hip and medially rotates the hip
Gracilis	Inferior pubic ramus	Medial proximal tibial shaft (pes anerine)	Adducts and flexes the hip; flexes and medially rotates the knee
Sartorius	Anterior superior iliac spine	Medial proximal tibial shaft (pes anserine)	Flexes, laterally rotates, and abducts the hip; medial and laterally rotates the knee when the knee is flexed.
Hamstrings Group			
Biceps femoris	Ischial tuberosity	Fibular head	Flexes the knee, laterally rotates the knee (when knee is flexed), extends the hip, medially rotates hip, posteriorly tilts the pelvis
Semitendonosis	Ischial tuberosity	Medial proximal tibial shaft (pes anserine)	Flexes the knee, medially rotates the knee (when knee is flexed), extends the hip, medially rotates hip, posteriorly tilts the pelvis
Semimembranosis	Ischial tuberosity	Medial condyle of the tibia	Flexes the knee, medially rotates the knee (when knee is flexed), extends the hip, medially rotates hip, posteriorly tilts the pelvis

TABLE 2-10 CONTINUED

Deep Six Hip Rotators

Muscle	Origin	Insertion	Action
Piriformis	Anterior surface of sacrum	Greater trochanter	Laterally rotates hip, abducts the hip when the hip is flexed
Quadratus femoris	Lateral border of ischial tuberosity	Intertrochanteric crest, between the greater and lesser trochanters	Laterally rotates the hip
Obturator internus	Obturator membrane and inferior surface of the obturator foramen	Medial surface of the greater trochanter	Laterally rotates the hip
Obturator externus	Superior and inferior rami of pubis	Trochanteric fossa of femur	Laterally rotates the hip
Gemellus superior	Ischial spine	Upper border of greater trochanter	Laterally rotates the hip
Gemellus inferior	Ischial tuberosity	Upper border of greater trochanter	Laterally rotates the hip

Quadriceps Group

Muscle	Origin	Insertion	Action
Rectus femoris	Anterior inferior iliac spine	Tibial tuberosity	Flexes the hip and extends the knee
Vastus lateralis	Linea aspera and gluteal tuberosity	Tibial tuberosity	Extends the knee
Vastus intermedialis	Anterior lateral femoral shaft	Tibial tuberosity	Extends the knee
Vastus medialis	Linea aspera	Tibial tuberosity	Extends the knee

Think about the action of the muscle to help you figure out its location. For example, for the toes to flex, it makes sense that the flexors be on the plantar aspect of the foot, whereas the extensors would be on the dorsal. Remember, muscles only pull; they never push. See Table 2-11 for muscles that move the ankle, foot, and toes (Figures 2-15, 2-16, and 2-17).

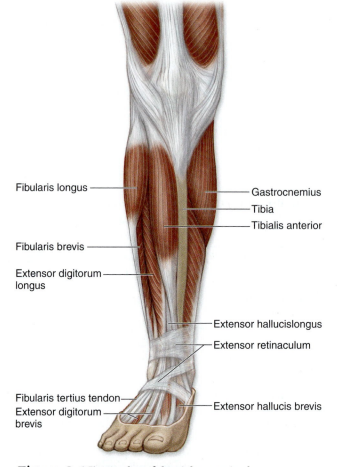

Fibularis longus

Gastrocnemius

Tibia

Tibialis anterior

Fibularis brevis

Extensor digitorum longus

Extensor hallucislongus

Extensor retinaculum

Fibularis tertius tendon

Extensor hallucis brevis

Extensor digitorum brevis

Figure 2-15 Muscles of the right anterior leg.

TABLE 2-11

At a Glance: Muscles That Move the Ankle, Foot, and Toes

Muscle	Origin	Insertion	Action
Tibialis anterior	Lateral tibial shaft and interosseous membrane	Base of the first metatarsal and cuneiform 1	Dorsiflexes the ankle and inverts the foot
Peroneus brevis (Fibularis brevis)	Lateral distal two-thirds of the fibular shaft	Base of fifth metatarsal	Everts the foot and plantar flexes the ankle
Peroneus longus (Fibularis longus)	Fibular head and lateral proximal two-thirds of the fibular shaft	Base of first metatarsal and cuneiform 1	Everts the foot and plantar flexes the ankle
Extensor digitorum longus and brevis	Longus: fibular head, proximal two-thirds of fibular shaft, and lateral condyle of the tibia.	Longus: middle halanges 2–5 and distal phalanges 2–5.	Extends digits 2–5 and dorsiflexes the ankle (longus only)
	Brevis: calcaneus	Brevis: tendons of extensor digitorum longus	
Gastrocnemius	Medial and lateral epicondyles of the femur	Calcaneus via the Achilles tendon femur	Plantar flexes the ankle and flexes the knee

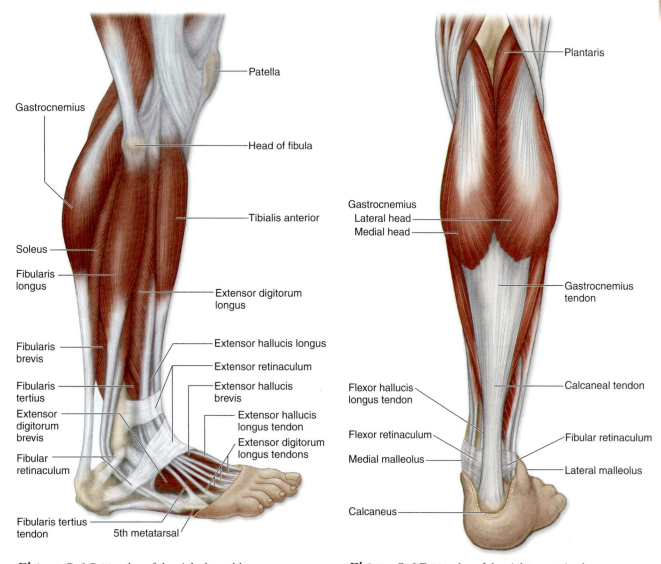

Figure 2-16 Muscles of the right lateral leg.

Figure 2-17 Muscles of the right posterior leg.

TABLE 2-11 CONTINUED

Muscle	Origin	Insertion	Action
Soleus	Superior posterior one-third of the fibular shaft and soleal line of the tibia	Calcaneus via the Achilles tendon	Plantar flexes the ankle
Flexor digitorum longus	Posterior tibial shaft-middle region	Distal phalanges 2–5	Flexes digits 2–5 at the DIP, PIP, MP joints and plantar flexes the ankle
Tibialis posterior	Posterior tibial shaft, posterior fibular shaft, and interosseous membrane	Navicular bone, third cuneiform, cuboid, and bases of metatarsals 2–4	Inverts the foot and plantar flexes the ankle
Flexor hallucis longus	Posterior fibular shaft	Distal phalanx of big toe	Flexes big toe, plantar flexes the ankle, inverts the foot, and supports the longitudinal arch
Extensor hallucis longus	Anterior fibular shaft, interosseous membrane	Distal phalanx of big toe	Extends the big toe and dorsiflexes the ankle

Joints

In order for muscles to move, we must have joints or articulations. The main types of joints in our bodies, as well as their description, movements, and examples, are listed below.

Fibrous: With this type of joint, articulating bones are fastened together by a thin layer of dense connective tissue. These joints do not move. An example is the sutures between bones of the skull.

Cartilaginous: In cartilaginous joints, articulating bones are connected by hyaline cartilage or fibrocartilage. They provide for limited movement, as when the back is bent or twisted. An example is the joints between the bodies of vertebrae and the symphysis pubis.

Synovial: With these joints, articulating bones are surrounded by a joint capsule of ligaments and synovial membranes; the ends of articulating bones are covered by hyaline cartilage and separated by synovial fluid. Several types are listed here:

1. **Ball-and-Socket**: The ball-shaped head of one bone articulates with the cup-shaped cavity of another bone. This movement occurs in all planes and rotations. Examples include the shoulder and hip.
2. **Condyloid**: The oval-shaped condyle of one bone articulates with the elliptical cavity of another. A variety of movements occur in different planes but no rotation. An example is the joints between the metacarpals and phalanges.
3. **Gliding**: Articulating surfaces are nearly flat or slightly curved which provides sliding or twisting movements. Gliding joints occur between various bones of the wrist and ankle, sacroiliac joint, joints between ribs two and the sternum and rib 7 and the sternum.
4. **Hinge**: The convex surface of one bone articulates with the concave surface of another. This makes flexion and extension possible, for example in the elbows, joints of phalanges, and knees.
5. **Pivot**: The cylindrical surface of one bone articulates with ring of bone and ligament, and rotates around a central axis. An example is the joint between the proximal ends of the radius and ulna.
6. **Saddle**: Articulating surfaces have both concave and convex regions; the surface of one bone fits the complementary surface of another, providing a variety of movements, for example, the joints between the carpal and metacarpal of the thumb.

Dermatomes

Dermatomes: These are a band-like unilateral patterns of peripheral nerves or an area or section supplied by a single spinal nerve (Figure 2-18).

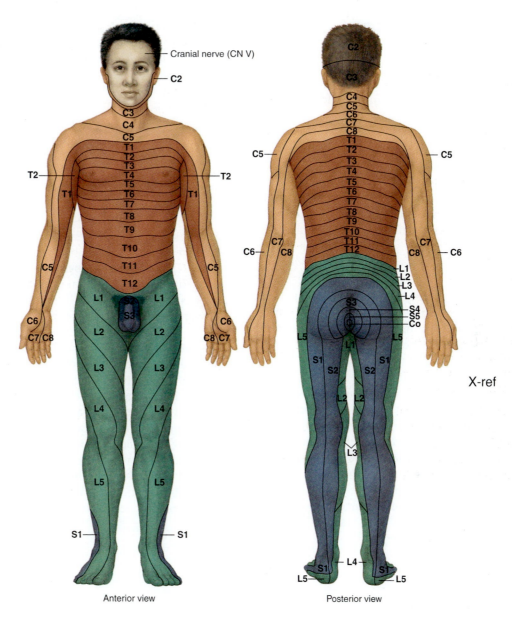

Figure 2-18 The dermatomes.

Nutrition

The Six Basic Nutrients

Six basic nutrients are needed in order for our bodies to survive.

Water: Water assists in many chemical functions, such as the formation of ATP. That is one reason we feel fatigued when we are dehydrated. Generally it is recommended to drink half your body weight in ounces of water daily; however, some disease situations contradict that. For example, those with congestive heart failure should follow the recommendations of their physician as to how much water they should drink.

Protein: Twelve to twenty percent of our diet should be made up of protein. Food sources include meats, poultry, beans, and legumes. Protein helps to repair and rebuild muscle. It does not *build* muscle as some think . . . exercise does!

Carbohydrates: Carbohydrates should make up fifty-five to sixty percent of our total diet. Carbohydrates help us to hold onto needed water. We have simple carbohydrates (refined sugars) which should be limited in our diet and complex carbohydrates (breads, pastas, cereals) that benefit our bodies and provide necessary energy. Carbohydrates are our primary fuel source—your brain uses twenty percent of all carbohydrates just to function. Some carbohydrates are high glycemic (good to eat after a bout of exercise to replace the fuel used), and others are mid/low glycemic (best to eat before a long bout of exercise).

Fats: Fats should make up no more than thirty percent of our total diet. Saturated fats are the bad fats that are generally solid at room temperature and should be no more than ten percent of our diet. Unsaturated fats are oils or liquid at room temperature and should make up no more that twenty percent of our caloric intake. Cholesterol falls into the fat category.

Vitamins: Vitamins have no caloric value but play a big role in a healthy diet. We have water soluble vitamins (B and C). If too much is ingested, our bodies expel the excess through the urine. Fat soluble vitamins (A, D, E, and K) are not expelled easily. Excesses are stored in the body fat and can create toxicity.

Minerals: Minerals are generally needed only in trace amounts. However, two minerals of concern to women are iron (important during the menstrual cycle years) and calcium (important during bone growing years of eleven to twenty-five and postmenopausal years). If supplemental iron or calcium is taken, it should be through a physician's recommendation.

Remember, our role in nutrition is to provide basic information, follow the FDA Food Guide Pyramid (Figure 2-19), and refer to a registered and licensed dietitian or the client's physician.

Memory Helper

There are two main types of cholesterol: HDL (high density lipoproteins) which are the good or "happy" cholesterol, and LDL (low density lipoprotein) which are the bad or "lousy" cholesterol.

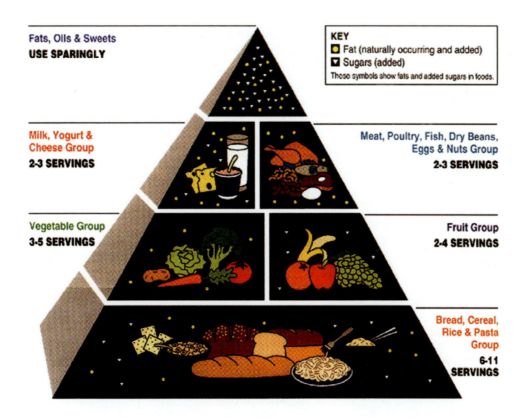

KEY
- ◘ Fat (naturally occurring and added)
- ▾ Sugars (added)

These symbols show fats and added sugars in foods.

Fats, Oils & Sweets
USE SPARINGLY

Milk, Yogurt & Cheese Group
2-3 SERVINGS

Meat, Poultry, Fish, Dry Beans, Eggs & Nuts Group
2-3 SERVINGS

Vegetable Group
3-5 SERVINGS

Fruit Group
2-4 SERVINGS

Bread, Cereal, Rice & Pasta Group
6-11 SERVINGS

Anatomy of MyPyramid

One size doesn't fit all

USDA's new MyPyramid symbolizes a personalized approach to healthy eating and physical activity. The symbol has been designed to be simple. It has been developed to remind consumers to make healthy food choices and to be active every day. The different parts of the symbol are described below.

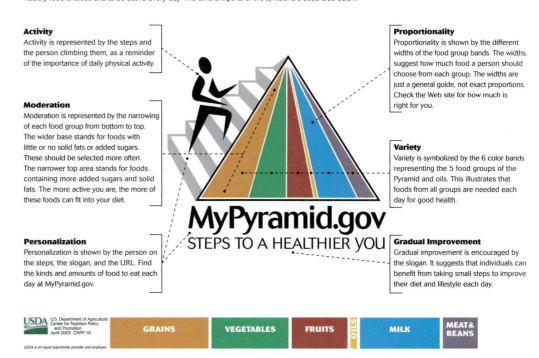

Activity
Activity is represented by the steps and the person climbing them, as a reminder of the importance of daily physical activity.

Moderation
Moderation is represented by the narrowing of each food group from bottom to top. The wider base stands for foods with little or no solid fats or added sugars. These should be selected more often. The narrower top area stands for foods containing more added sugars and solid fats. The more active you are, the more of these foods can fit into your diet.

Personalization
Personalization is shown by the person on the steps, the slogan, and the URL. Find the kinds and amounts of food to eat each day at MyPyramid.gov.

Proportionality
Proportionality is shown by the different widths of the food group bands. The widths suggest how much food a person should choose from each group. The widths are just a general guide, not exact proportions. Check the Web site for how much is right for you.

Variety
Variety is symbolized by the 6 color bands representing the 5 food groups of the Pyramid and oils. This illustrates that foods from all groups are needed each day for good health.

Gradual Improvement
Gradual improvement is encouraged by the slogan. It suggests that individuals can benefit from taking small steps to improve their diet and lifestyle each day.

MyPyramid.gov
STEPS TO A HEALTHIER YOU

USDA U.S. Department of Agriculture
Center for Nutrition Policy and Promotion
April 2005 CNPP-16

USDA is an equal opportunity provider and employer.

GRAINS   VEGETABLES   FRUITS   OILS   MILK   MEAT & BEANS

Figure 2-19 The FDA Food Guide Pyramid. In 2005, the FDA announced a new food pyramid, seen here alongside the previous pyramid, which you will need to know for your exam.

Strategies to Success

Test-Taking Skills

No tricks, just focus!

Always read all of the responses to a question before answering. If you choose an answer too quickly, you might miss the best answer. Don't make assumptions about the questions and how the writer of the question might be trying to trick you. Use only the information provided in the question, and choose the best answer based on your knowledge of the subject.

*Some questions are not directly addressed in this chapter, but are meant to act as a general review of subjects studied in various school curriculums.

Questions

NCETM (26%) NCETMB (26%)

1. The type of stretching where temporary lengthening of the muscle is the goal is called
   A. stretch reflex.
   B. elastic elongation.
   C. plastic elongation.
   D. post-event stretch.

2. When the anterior superior iliac spine (ASIS) is lower than the posterior superior iliac spine (PSIS) in postural analysis, this means
   A. an anterior pelvic tilt.
   B. a posterior pelvic tilt.
   C. a high hip.
   D. None of the above are correct.

3. The insertion of the sternocleidomastoid is
   A. manubrium.
   B. medial clavicle.
   C. sternum.
   D. mastoid process.

4. Two muscles that insert on rib 1 are
   A. posterior scalenes and anterior scalenes.
   B. middle scalenes and anterior scalenes.

C. posterior scalenes and sternocleidomastoid.
D. posterior scalenes only.

5. The muscle that is also known as the "six pack" is the
   A. external oblique.
   B. rectus abdominus.
   C. internal oblique.
   D. transverse abdominus.

6. The insertion for the triceps brachii is
   A. radial tuberosity.
   B. supraglenoid fossa.
   C. coracoid process.
   D. olecranon process.

7. External rotators of the shoulder are
   A. supraspinatus and teres minor.
   B. subscapularis and supraspinatus.
   C. teres major and infraspinatus.
   D. teres minor and infraspinatus.

8. A band of connective tissue that wraps around tendons is called
   A. retinaculum.
   B. aponeurosis.
   C. fascia.
   D. myocardium.

9. If your client has an anterior pelvic tilt, this means that the
   A. hamstrings are tight and the rectus femoris is stretched.
   B. rectus femoris is tight and the biceps femoris is stretched.
   C. biceps femoris is tight and the rectus femoris is stretched.
   D. hamstrings are tight and the iliopsoas is stretched.

10. If your client has an exaggerated outward curve of the thoracic spine, he or she is
    A. kyphotic.
    B. lordotic.
    C. sway back.
    D. scolitic.

11. Your client is internally rotated at the shoulders. This means you need to focus on what muscles in his or her massage session?
    A. infraspinatus and teres minor
    B. latissimus dorsi and teres minor
    C. supraspinatus and latissimus dorsi
    D. subscapularis and latissimus dorsi

12. Which of the following represents poor body mechanics or positioning?
    A. bending at the waist to increase leverage
    B. hands and arms relaxed to the side of the body
    C. knees slightly bent with weight evenly distributed on both feet
    D. shoulders relaxed

13. The anterior cruciate ligament attaches the
    A. humerus to the radius.
    B. anterior side of each vertebrae.
    C. femur and the tibia.
    D. fibula and the femur.

14. What type of muscle is NOT striated?
    A. visceral
    B. cardiac
    C. mylineated
    D. skeletal

15. The vastus lateralis muscle inserts at the
    A. posterior medial tibial condyle.
    B. tibial tuberosity.
    C. posterior lateral tibial condyle.
    D. ischial tuberosity.

16. The nerve endings located in the tendon that protect the tendon and muscle from over-contracting and are over-ridden in fight or flight are called
    A. Golgi tendons.
    B. muscle spindles.
    C. proprioceptors.
    D. stretch reflex.

17. The hip joint is made up of
    A. the femur and infraglenoid fossa.
    B. the femur and the pubic symphysis.
    C. the femur and the acetabulum.
    D. the femur and the ischium.

18. The medial malleolus is the distal end of the
    A. radius.
    B. ulna.
    C. tibia.
    D. fibula.

19. The muscles that perform mastication are the
    A. masseter, medial pterygoid, lateral pterygoid, and temporalis.
    B. masseter, suprahyoid, platysma, and temporalis.
    C. masseter, omohyoid, temporalis, and platysma.
    D. masseter, medial pterygoid, lateral ptery-goid, and platysma.

20. The deep six hip rotators include all of the following except
    A. gemellus superior.
    B. gemellus interior.
    C. quadratus femoris.
    D. obturator internus.

21. Which of the following muscles does NOT attach to the os coxae?
    A. internal oblique
    B. sartorius
    C. vastus lateralis
    D. semimembranosus

22. What are the three muscles that attach to the coracoid process?
    A. pectoralis minor, biceps brachii, and coracobrachialis
    B. pectoralis major, biceps brachii, and coracobrachialis
    C. pectoralis major, brachialis, and coracobrachialis
    D. pectoralis minor, brachialis, and coracobrachialis

23. The tibialis anterior muscle attaches at the base of the
    A. first metatarsal and dorsiflexes the foot.
    B. first metatarsal and plantar flexes the foot.
    C. fifth metatarsal and dorsiflexes the foot.
    D. fifth metatarsal and plantar flexes the foot.

24. Another name for a hairline fracture is a
    A. stress fracture.
    B. comminuted fracture.
    C. compression fracture.
    D. compound fracture.

25. The joint type that allows for the most range of motion is the
    A. diarthroses.
    B. synchondrosis.
    C. sutured.
    D. fibrous.

26. The ligament that helps support the femur–tibia joint is the
    A. deltoid ligament.
    B. anterior cruciate ligament.
    C. glenoid labrum.
    D. femoral acetabulum ligament.

27. Your client has hurt his or her ankle. It is very swollen and discolored. He or she may have what type of injury?
    A. a third degree sprain
    B. a third degree strain
    C. a first degree sprain
    D. a first degree strain

28. A muscle that when tight can cause sciatica and externally rotate the hip is the
    A. gluteus maximus.
    B. gluteus minimus.
    C. iliopsoas.
    D. piriformis.

29. A muscle that flexes the knee and extends the hip is the
    A. biceps femoris.
    B. rectus femoris.
    C. vastus lateralis.
    D. gluteus maximus.

30. All of the following are rotator cuff muscles except the
    A. teres minor.
    B. teres major.
    C. subscapularis.
    D. supraspinatus.

31. The origin of the deltoid muscle is the
    A. lateral one-third of clavicle, acromion process, and crest of scapular spine.
    B. medial one-third of clavicle, acromion process, and crest of scapular spine.
    C. lateral one-third of clavicle, glenoid fossa, and crest of scapular spine.
    D. deltoid tuberosity.

32. What nerve innervates the trapezius?
    A. spinal accessory
    B. long thoracic
    C. pectoral nerve
    D. trapezius nerve

33. What is the insertion of the long head of the triceps?
    A. olecranon process
    B. infraglenoid fossa
    C. supraglenoid fossa
    D. coracoid process

34. What muscles flex the elbow?
    A. triceps and anconeus
    B. brachialis, biceps brachii, and supinator
    C. brachioradialis, supinator, and coracobrachialis
    D. pronator teres, brachioradialis, and brachialis

35. What muscles extend the elbow?
    A. triceps and anconeus
    B. brachialis, biceps, and supinator

C. brachioradialis, supinator, and coracobrachialis
D. pronator teres, brachioradialis, and brachialis

36. What are the boundaries/borders of the cubital fossa?
    A. semitendonosis, sartorius, and biceps femoris.
    B. brachioradialis, pronator teres, and the line between the humeral epicondyles.
    C. adductor magnus, gracilis, and adductor brevis.
    D. None of the above are correct.

37. What two muscles are connected by the broad epicranial aponeurosis?
    A. temporalis and occipitalis
    B. temporalis and frontalis
    C. frontalis and occipitalis
    D. frontalis and masseter

38. The meeting of the ilium, ischium, and pubis forms the
    A. pubis symphysis.
    B. ischial tuberosity.
    C. ramus.
    D. acetabulum.

39. The ligaments that help prevent rotation of the knee are the
    A. anterior cruciate and the posterior cruciate.
    B. medial collateral and the lateral collateral.
    C. the inferior cruciate and the superior cruciate.
    D. the patellar ligament.

40. Which specific joint in the body is the most mobile?
    A. the shoulder
    B. the hip
    C. the metacarpal-phalange
    D. the wrist

41. What are the major actions of the peroneus longus and brevis?
    A. inversion and dorsiflexion of the foot
    B. inversion and plantarflexion of the foot
    C. eversion and plantar flexion of the foot
    D. eversion and dorsiflexion of the foot

42. The mouth opens in a hinge-like motion due to which joint?
    A. temporopteygoid joint
    B. maxilla–mandibular joint
    C. ethmoid–sphenoid joint
    D. temporomandibular joint

43. Paresthesia is a medical term for
    A. paralysis.
    B. prickly, tingling feeling in a limb.
    C. an abnormal opening.
    D. excessive thirst.

44. How many types of synovial joints are there?
    A. three
    B. four
    C. five
    D. six

45. Which of the following is NOT one of the carpal bones?
    A. hamate
    B. scaphoid
    C. lunate
    D. cuneiform

46. All of the following muscles form the tendon of the ligamentum patellae except
    A. rectus femoris.
    B. vastus lateralis.
    C. biceps femoris.
    D. vastus intermedialis.

47. The weight-bearing part of the foot is
    A. calcaneus.
    B. heads of metatarsal bones one and five.
    C. heads of metatarsal bones one through five.
    D. Both A and B are correct.

48. The border of the posterior triangle of the neck are all of the following except
    A. middle one-third of the clavicle.
    B. sternocleidomastoid.
    C. latissimus dorsi.
    D. trapezius.

49. Hinge joints allow what type of movements?
    A. abduction and adduction
    B. medial and lateral rotation
    C. flexion and extension
    D. circumduction

50. The cartilage that surrounds and protects the ends of long bones is called
    A. fibrocartilage.
    B. hyaline cartilage.
    C. periosteum.
    D. None of the above are correct.

51. The class of joints where bones or cartilage are joined only by fibrous tissue are called
    A. fibrous.
    B. syndesmosis.
    C. hinge.
    D. condylar.

52. The bony projection on C2 is called the
    A. axis.
    B. atlas.
    C. odontoid.
    D. None of the above are correct.

53. Movement between C1 and the skull is
    A. flexion/extension.
    B. lateral flexion.
    C. rotation.
    D. No movement occurs here.

54. Movement between C1 and C2 is
    A. flexion/extension.
    B. lateral flexion.
    C. rotation.
    D. No movement occurs here.

55. What bone is on the anterior neck?
    A. thyroid
    B. cricoid
    C. hyoid
    D. thymus

56. All of the following muscles form the border of the popliteal fossa except
    A. biceps femoris.
    B. gastrocnemius.
    C. semimembranosus.
    D. gracilis.

57. Which of the following is a rounded bony landmark that is for articulation?
    A. epicondyle
    B. tuberosity
    C. condyle
    D. fossa

58. What structure in the popliteal fossa makes this area an endangerment site?
    A. sciatic nerve
    B. tibial nerve
    C. the posterior thigh nerve
    D. peroneal nerve

59. What anatomical structure should be avoided when massaging around the sartorius and adductor longus muscles?
    A. sciatic nerve
    B. popliteal artery
    C. inferior vena cava
    D. femoral artery

60. All of the following are general effects of heat except
    A. increased blood flow.
    B. decreased metabolic rate.
    C. increased pulse rate.
    D. dialation of peripheral blood vessels.

61. Which of the following is considered an ellipsoidal joint?
    A. wrist
    B. elbow
    C. knee
    D. hip

62. Your client has had an inversion ankle sprain. The muscle that should be strengthened is the
    A. tibialis anterior.
    B. posterior tibalis.
    C. gastrocnemius.
    D. peroneus longus.

63. The carotid sinus is located
    A. posterior neck triangle.
    B. anterior neck triangle.
    C. brachial plexus area.
    D. deltopectoral area.

64. Ligaments are
    A. slow to heal.
    B. receive poor blood supply.
    C. attach bone to bone.
    D. All of the above are correct.

65. The lubricating fluid that is found in moveable joints is called
    A. serous fluid.
    B. synovial fluid.
    C. arthropometric fluid.
    D. diarthrotic fluid.

66. The anterior superior iliac spine is located on which bone?
    A. vertebrae
    B. hyoid
    C. ischium
    D. ilium

67. This joint allows pronation and supination of the hand
    A. radioulnar.
    B. intercarpal.
    C. radiocarpal.
    D. ulnarcarpal.

68. The abdominal muscle group includes all of the following except
    A. rectus femoris.
    B. rectus abdominus.
    C. internal oblique.
    D. external oblique.

69. The coranoid process is located on the
    A. radius.
    B. ulna.
    C. scapula.
    D. clavicle.

70. The most abundant and widely distributed tissue of the body is
    A. connective tissue.
    B. epithelial tissue.
    C. serous tissue.
    D. tendons.

71. Which muscle is the only muscle that moves the head but does not attach to any vertebrae?
    A. scalenes
    B. trapezius
    C. splenius capitus
    D. sternocleidomastoid

72. The muscle that can entrap the brachial nerve, artery, and vein is pectoralis minor and
    A. SCM.
    B. scalenes.
    C. spenius capitus.
    D. None of the above are correct.

73. Which of the following is not a function of the muscular system?
    A. creating external and internal movement
    B. maintaining posture
    C. production of heat
    D. exchange of gases

74. The ischial tuberosity is located on the
    A. ischium.
    B. ilium.
    C. sacrum.
    D. pubic bone.

75. The largest joint in the body
    A. shoulder.
    B. knee.
    C. hip.
    D. elbow.

76. The sensory receptors stimulated by both tension and excessive stretch and activated an inhibitory response in the motor neuron are called
    A. muscle spindles.
    B. golgi tendons.
    C. baroreceptors.
    D. proprioceptors.

77. Which muscle crosses two joints?
    A. anconeus
    B. brachialis
    C. gastrocnemius
    D. soleus

78. The function of ligaments is
    A. to provide mobility.
    B. to stabilize the joint.
    C. to cushion.
    D. None of the above are correct.

79. The sciatic nerve can be compressed and irritated when which muscle is tight?
    A. biceps femoris
    B. rectus abdominus
    C. adductor magnus
    D. piriformis

80. The type of movement that occurs at the distal radioulnar joint is
    A. gliding.
    B. abduction.
    C. circumduction.
    D. rotation.

81. Your client's lower back hurts when he or she lies flat. The muscles that might be tight would be
    A. iliopsoas and rectus femoris.
    B. iliopsoas and biceps femoris.
    C. quadratus femoris and rectus femoris.
    D. quadratus lumborum and biceps femoris.

82. Winged scapula is weakness in which muscle?
    A. supraspinatus
    B. infraspinatus
    C. serratus anterior
    D. subscaularis

83. From the anatomical position, the semitendonosis is immediately superficial to the
    A. biceps femoris.
    B. semimembranosus.
    C. rectus femoris.
    D. plantaris.

84. Fats are classified as
    A. solid or liquid.
    B. saturated or unsaturated.
    C. water soluble or fat soluble.
    D. Both A and B are correct.

85. The largest sesamoid bone in the body is the
    A. ischial tuberosity.
    B. xiphoid process.
    C. patella.
    D. malleolus.

86. The muscles used in forced expiration are
    A. diaphragm and abdominals.
    B. abdominals.
    C. internal and external intercostals.
    D. external intercostals and levator scapula.

87. The joint that is generally involved in a shoulder separation is the
    A. glenohumeral.
    B. acromioclavicular.
    C. coracoid-humeral.
    D. humeral-scapular.

88. Migraine headaches are generally
    A. tension headaches.
    B. vascular headaches.
    C. phantom headaches.
    D. All of the above are correct.

89. A tough, dense material that has the greatest tensile strength and is found in the intervertebral disks is
    A. elastic cartilage.
    B. fibrocartilage.
    C. hyaline cartilage.
    D. osseous cartilage.

90. This is referred to as the yes–yes joint
    A. atlanto–occipital joint.
    B. atlantoaxial joint.
    C. acromioclavicular joint.
    D. the occipital–temporal joint.

91. The bones of the vertebral column, skull, hyoid, and pelvis make up the
    A. appendicular skeleton.
    B. diarthrotic skeleton.
    C. axial skeleton.
    D. axis skeleton.

92. The pes anserine is made up of all of the following muscles except
    A. sartorius.
    B. semimembranosus.
    C. gracilis.
    D. semitendonosis.

93. Golfer's elbow is irritation on the
    A. lateral epicondyle.
    B. medial epicondyle.
    C. olecranon process.
    D. radial tuberosity.

94. This bone is also known as the atlas
    A. C2.
    B. C1.
    C. L2.
    D. S1.

95. Slow, light, and rhythmic movements are soothing to the nerves because they produce a low level of excitement to the nervous system, whereas vigorous movements
    A. stimulate the parasympathetic nervous system.
    B. decrease synaptic transmission.
    C. excite nociceptors.
    D. stimulate the sympathetic nervous system.

96. The receptors for vibration and touch are called the
    A. proproceptors.
    B. nociceptors.
    C. mechanoreceptors.
    D. noreceptors.

97. First stages of healing result in
    A. increased fibrin production.
    B. histamine release.

C. redness of skin.
D. collagen remodeling.

98. Functions of the connective tissue include all of the following except
    A. nutrient transportation.
    B. defense against disease.
    C. clotting mechanisms.
    D. neural transport.

99. Fluid found in all diarthrotic joints is
    A. synovial.
    B. serous.
    C. tissue.
    D. visceral.

100. Nerve endings that are pressure sensitive and respond to skin displacement are
    A. free nerve endings.
    B. Meissner's corpuscles.
    C. Pacinian's corpuscles.
    D. Krause's end bulbs.

101. What layer of connective tissue wraps around the entire muscle?
    A. endomysium
    B. ectomysium
    C. perimysium
    D. epimysium

102. Which bones are not one of the five classifications?
    A. long
    B. short
    C. regular
    D. sesmoid

103. Certain massage strokes create minute muscle contractions by
    A. increasing golgi tendon response.
    B. increasing muscle spindle activity.
    C. increasing lymph flow.
    D. stimulation of the myosin.

104. Cartilage that is found on the tip of the nose and the lobes of the ears is called
    A. fibrocartilage.
    B. hyaline cartilage.
    C. meniscus.
    D. elastic cartilage.

105. Carbohydrates are classified as
    A. solid or liquid.
    B. mono-, di-, tri-, and polysaccharides.
    C. water soluble or fat soluble.
    D. saturated or unsaturated.

106. All of the following are types of connective tissue except
    A. blood.
    B. cartilage.
    C. ligaments.
    D. organs.

107. All of the following are functions of adipose tissue except
    A. protection.
    B. thermal heat.
    C. movement.
    D. insulation.

108. The ability of a muscle to return to its original shape after being stretched is known as
    A. irritability.
    B. contractibility.
    C. plastic elongation.
    D. PNF.

109. The three main types of connective tissue of the skeletal system are all of the following except
    A. ligaments.
    B. joint capsule.
    C. cartilage.
    D. tendons.

110. The common origin of the hamstrings is the
    A. medial tibal condyle.
    B. lateral tibal condyle.
    C. PSIS.
    D. ischial tuberosity.

111. Which area of the spine has the most vertebrae?
    A. cervical
    B. thoracic
    C. lumbar
    D. sacral

112. The name of the upper jaw bone is the
    A. zygomatic.
    B. masseter.
    C. mandible.
    D. maxilla.

113. Receptors responding to air vibrations or sound waves are the
    A. mechanoreceptors.
    B. chemoreceptors.
    C. photoreceptors.
    D. nociceptors.

114. Lumbricles are located in the
    A. hands.
    B. feet.
    C. lumbar vertebrae.
    D. Both A and B are correct.

115. Small canals found in the bone that help to nourish it are called
    A. Pacinian canals.
    B. Haversian canals.
    C. Meissner canals.
    D. marrow.

116. The capitulum of the humerus articulates with
    A. lateral condyles of the humerus.
    B. olecranon.
    C. ulnar head.
    D. radial head.

117. The sternum articulates with how many ribs?
    A. twelve pairs
    B. six pairs
    C. seven pairs
    D. five pairs

118. The greater amount of rotation in the spine occurs in the
    A. thoracic region.
    B. cervical region.
    C. lumbar region.
    D. sacral region.

119. Which bone is not in the distal row of the carpals?
    A. capitate
    B. hamate
    C. lunate
    D. trapezoid

120. What are the major actions of the peroneus longus and brevis?
    A. Inversion and dorsiflexion of the foot
    B. Inversion and plantar flexion of the foot
    C. Eversion and plantar flexion of the foot
    D. Eversion and dorsiflexion of the foot

121. Your client has an anterior pelvic tilt. In addition to the quads and iliopsoas, what other muscle would tilt the pelvis anteriorly if tight?
    A. gluteus maximus
    B. piriformis
    C. biceps femoris
    D. Tensor fascia latae/ITB

122. The quadriceps muscles are all of the following except
    A. vastus lateralis.
    B. rectus femoris.
    C. biceps femoris.
    D. vastus intermedialis.

123. What is the largest muscle in the body?
    A. sartorius
    B. gluteus maximus
    C. quadriceps
    D. abdominas

124. When the quads receive information to contract and the hamstrings receive information to relax, this is known as
    A. muscle tone.
    B. atrophy.
    C. reciprocal inhibition.
    D. sliding filament theory.

125. The type of heat illness that is a medical emergency is
    A. heat cramps.
    B. hypothermia.
    C. heat stroke.
    D. heat exhaustion.

126. If your client has an exaggerated outward curve of the thoracic spine, he or she is
    A. kyphotic.
    B. lordotic.
    C. sway back.
    D. scoliotic.

127. Another term for pes planus is
    A. flat feet.
    B. high arches.
    C. lost transverse arch.
    D. None of the above are correct.

128. The pear-shaped sac located on the right side of the body that stores bile is called the
    A. liver.
    B. pancreas.
    C. gallbladder.
    D. stomach.

129. A client with lordosis may experience a reduction in low back discomfort if a pillow is placed under the
    A. abdomen in the prone position.
    B. chest in the prone position.
    C. pelvis in the prone position.
    D. None of the above are correct.

130. Stretching can be done _____ by the therapist with no assistance from the client or _____ by the client with no assistance from the therapist.
    A. passively; actively
    B. actively; passively
    C. PNF; MET
    D. ballistically; statically

131. A muscle synergistic to the biceps brachii is the
    A. brachialis.
    B. coracobrachialis.
    C. brachioradialis.
    D. triceps.

132. Repetitive motion injuries are caused by
    A. repeated flexing and extending of a joint against resistance.
    B. normal daily activities.
    C. manual manipulation of tools.
    D. Both A and C are correct.

133. When the hamstrings are acting as an antagonist, the movement is
    A. hip extension.
    B. knee extension.
    C. knee flexion.
    D. Both A and C are correct.

134. Which muscle is not a part of the shoulder girdle group?
    A. pectoralis minor
    B. trapezius
    C. deltoid
    D. bicep brachii

135. Where is the least amount of movement in the spine?
    A. C3–C6
    B. T4–T6
    C. T1–T3
    D. L4–L5

136. The muscle that initiates shoulder abduction is
    A. the medial deltoid.
    B. supraspinatus.
    C. subscapularis.
    D. latissimus dorsi.

137. Plantar fasciitis can be caused by all of the following except
    A. old shoes.
    B. high arches.
    C. low arches.
    D. tight peroneals.

138. When slowly sitting down in a chair, how are muscles being worked?
    A. hamstrings concentrically
    B. quadriceps eccentrically
    C. gluteals concentrically
    D. all of the above

139. Which muscle abducts the hip?
    A. gluteus maximus
    B. gluteus medius
    C. hamstrings
    D. gracilis

140. Another name for the cheek bone is the
    A. temporalis bone.
    B. ethmoid bone.
    C. zygomatic bone.
    D. pterygoid.

141. The ITB is _____ to the gracilis.
    A. medial
    B. lateral
    C. superior
    D. proximal

142. The function of the masseter muscle is to
    A. extend the jaw.
    B. retract the jaw.
    C. open the jaw.
    D. close the jaw.

143. Which muscle helps us to smile?
    A. zygomaticus
    B. masseter
    C. orbicularis oris
    D. temporalis

144. When the serratus anterior contracts, what movement takes place?
    A. scapular retraction
    B. scapular protraction
    C. scapular elevation
    D. scapular depression

145. Which muscle depresses the ribs?
    A. scalenes
    B. pectoralis minor
    C. internal intercostals
    D. external intercostals

146. Which muscle is also known as the "hip hiker"?
    A. quadratus femoris
    B. quadratus lumborum
    C. quadratus teres
    D. latissimus dorsi

147. The trapezius is _____ to the rhomboids.
    A. superficial
    B. deep
    C. medial
    D. superior

148. In placing the bolster under the ankle when the client is prone, you are preventing excessive
    A. dorsiflexion of the ankle.
    B. flexion of the knee.
    C. plantar flexion.
    D. None of the above are correct.

149. The metacarpals are _____ to the carpals.
    A. proximal
    B. distal
    C. medial
    D. lateral

150. Muscles that adduct the femur include all of the following except
    A. adductor magnus.
    B. gracilis.
    C. sartorius.
    D. pectineus.

151. In lordosis, which muscles would be weakened?
    A. quadriceps
    B. hamstrings
    C. iliopsoas
    D. quadratus lumborum

152. When the body is standing with the hands supinated, arms slightly abducted, and feet facing forward, this is known as the
    A. Eastern anatomical position.
    B. Northern anatomical position.
    C. Western anatomical position.
    D. essential medical position.

153. With your client's elbow bent to ninety degrees, you apply resistance as he pulls his hand towards the navel. Pain is felt. This would be inflammation of
    A. latissimus dorsi.
    B. pectoralis major.
    C. subscapularis.
    D. All of the above are correct.

154. The most common ankle sprain is the inversion sprain because
    A. the medial malleolus is lower on the medial side.
    B. because the stronger ligaments are on the lateral side of the ankle.
    C. because the lateral malleolus is lower on the lateral side.
    D. because talo fibular ligament is not in a mechanically strong place.

155. You are performing a push-up. You get about halfway off the floor and cannot push the rest of the way up. You struggle to go up, but you won't move. What type of muscle contraction is occurring on the biceps brachii?
    A. isometric
    B. isotonic
    C. eccentric
    D. concentric

156. Your client states he or she was running outdoors, planted his or her foot and twisted the knee which is now painful and swollen. What structure may be damaged?
    A. the ACL
    B. the PCL
    C. the MCL
    D. the patellar tendon

157. Which rotator cuff muscle does not rotate the humerus?
    A. supraspinatus
    B. infraspinatus
    C. teres minor
    D. subscapularis

158. Which end of the muscle has the most movement?
    A. the ligament
    B. the insertion
    C. the origin
    D. none of the above

159. The "kissing" muscle is the
    A. buccinator.
    B. masster.
    C. orbicularis oris.
    D. platysma.

160. Which of the following is not part of the iliopsoas muscle?
    A. iliacus
    B. psoas major
    C. psoas minor
    D. iliacus major

161. If the erector spinae is contracted bilaterally, this would result in
    A. scoliosis.
    B. kyphosis.
    C. rotation.
    D. lordosis.

162. If a client has torn his or her supraspinatus muscle, he or she will not be able to
    A. open a door.
    B. hold his or her arm out to the side.
    C. push a grocery cart.
    D. None of the above are correct.

163. If a client has drop foot, the muscle affected is
    A. gastrocnemius.
    B. soleus.
    C. anterior tibialis.
    D. peroneals.

164. A concentric contraction of the biceps femoris results in
    A. hip extension.
    B. hip flexion.
    C. knee extension.
    D. internal hip rotatation.

165. A concentric contraction of the biceps brachii results in
    A. elbow extension.
    B. shoulder extension.
    C. shoulder adduction.
    D. elbow flexion.

166. When standing and performing trunk flexion, the primary muscle mover is
    A. rectus abdominus.
    B. internal/external oblique.
    C. erector spinae eccentrically.
    D. None of the above are correct.

167. In order to strengthen anterior tibialis, your client can
    A. walk on his or her heels only.
    B. walk on his or her toes.
    C. perform heel raises.
    D. All of the above are correct.

168. Thrusting the lower jaw forward is called
    A. protraction.
    B. retraction.
    C. elevation.
    D. depression.

169. The three muscles that cause internal shoulder rotation include all of the following except
    A. infraspinatus.
    B. latissimus dorsi.
    C. pectoralis major.
    D. subscapularis.

170. Starches belong to which basic nutrient group?
    A. proteins
    B. fats
    C. meats
    D. carbohydrates

171. When the sole of the foot is turned outward, this is called
    A. inversion.
    B. eversion.
    C. pronatiaon.
    D. supination.

172. Which muscle flexes the knee and attaches to the fibula?
    A. biceps femoris
    B. rectus femoris
    C. semitendonosis
    D. semimembranosis

173. What muscle initiates walking?
    A. iliopsoas
    B. vastus lateralis
    C. vastus medialis
    D. hamstrings

174. Your client is having trouble laterally flexing his or her head. Which muscle is not involved?
    A. sternocleidomastoid
    B. splenius capitus
    C. cervical lamina
    D. splenius cervicus

175. When stepping down off a curb, what kind of contraction is occuring?
    A. concentric on the quads
    B. eccentric on the quads
    C. concentric on the hamstrings
    D. eccentric on the hamstrings

176. The three muscles of the erector spinae in order from most lateral to most medial are
    A. longissimus, spinalis, and iliocostalis.
    B. spinalis, iliocostalis, and longissimus.
    C. iliocostalis, spinalis, and longissimus.
    D. iliocostalis, longissimus, and spinalis.

177. The most distal bones of the foot are called
    A. tarsals.
    B. phalanges.
    C. carpals.
    D. metatarsals.

178. Another term for scapular adduction is
    A. horizontal shoulder flexion.
    B. protraction.
    C. retraction.
    D. extension.

179. In performing a squat, the stabilizer would be
    A. gastrocnemius/soleus.
    B. rectus abdominus.
    C. iliopsoas.
    D. hamstrings.

180. The fat soluble vitamins include all of the following except
    A. A.
    B. E.
    C. B.
    D. K.

181. The basic nutrients include the following except
    A. carbohydrates.
    B. cholesterol.
    C. fats.
    D. protein.

182. Guidelines to consider when using herbs or supplements include
    A. more is not necessarily better.
    B. ask friends their dosage since one dosage is suitable for all.
    C. if the dosage does not work quickly, change your dosage.
    D. All of the above are correct.

183. An excellent natural antibiotic is
    A. basil.
    B. jojoba.
    C. licorice.
    D. garlic.

184. The appropriate amount of carbohydrates in the diet according to the American Dietetic Association (ADA) is
    A. twelve to twenty percent.
    B. forty-five to sixty-five percent.
    C. ten to twenty percent.
    D. more than thirty percent.

185. The most unhealthy fats are called
    A. unsaturated.
    B. HDL.
    C. saturated.
    D. LDL.

186. High glycemic foods are
    A. foods that are low in sugar.
    B. foods that are high in sugar.
    C. foods best eaten before a long bout of exercise.
    D. Both A and C are correct.

187. _____ are one of the six basic nutrients with no caloric value that are needed in the body in small (trace) amounts.
    A. Vitamins
    B. Proteins
    C. Minerals
    D. Fats

188. Vitamins that can be harmful to the body if taken in huge amounts are called
    A. fat soluble.
    B. water soluble.
    C. vitamin C.
    D. vitamin B.

189. One gram of fat equals _____ calories.
    A. four
    B. seven
    C. nine
    D. twelve

190. The glucose amount that is ideal in sports drinks is
    A. more than ten percent.
    B. ten to twelve percent.
    C. less than five percent.
    D. six to eight percent.

191. Which vitamin best helps the body to absorb calcium?
    A. vitamin A
    B. vitamin B
    C. vitamin C
    D. vitamin D

192. Which mineral is a concern for those taking diuretics because it tends to be flushed out of the body easier?
    A. zinc
    B. potassium
    C. calcium
    D. chromium

193. Minerals that assist in the production of ATP are
    A. chromium.
    B. creatine.
    C. potassium.
    D. Both A and B are correct.

194. A plant that is excellent to use on minor burns is
    A. aloe vera.
    B. licorice.
    C. ivy.
    D. wild cherry bark.

195. The following are true concerning sugar except
    A. can improve the immune system.
    B. contributes to obesity.
    C. can increase the risk of osteoporosis.
    D. can produce an acidic stomach.

Answers and Explanations

NCETM (26%) NCETMB (26%)

1. **B** Remember, rubber bands are elastic and temporarily lengthen before going back to their original length. Plastic elongation is more permanent, like the plastic bottle that will maintain its shape. Therefore, elastic elongation is temporary and more for pre-event or pre-exercise with the goal of preparing you for exertional movement. Plastic elongation stretch is for post-exercise to help improve, in a more permanent way, flexibility.

2. **A** Think of your pelvis as a basin of water. Tilt the basin downward in the front, and the water spills out in front. If the pelvis does the same movement, this is an anterior pelvic tilt. In this case, the anterior superior iliac spine is tilted down or lower in front than the posterior iliac spine in back. This is commonly seen in people whose pants are higher in the back on the waist and low in front on the waist.

3. **D** The origin is the medial clavicle and the manubrium of the sternum. The insertion, which is the question, is the mastoid process.

4. **B** The posterior scalenes attaches to rib 2; the sternocleidomastoid attaches to the clavicle and the sternum, not to the ribs.

5. **B** When someone is very toned with low body fat, the rectus abdominus gives the appearance of separate little muscle bulges, thus the name "six pack."

6. **D** The other three answer choices listed are origins and insertions for the biceps brachii.

7. **D** Remember the EX in external, the I in infraspinatus, and the T in teres minor, and you have EXIT.

8. **A** Aponeurosis is a flat, broad tendon that attaches skeletal muscle to bone, to another muscle, or to skin; myocardium is the muscle of the heart; fascia is the lining around muscles, blood vessels, and nerves that connects them to surrounding tissue to hold them in place.

9. **B** An anterior pelvic tilt means muscles attaching to the anterior side of the pelvis are pulling it downward in the front (the ASIS is lower than the PSIS). Therefore muscles attaching to the ASIS and the AIIS are tight; muscles attaching to the PSIS, ischial tuberosity will be stretched.

10. **A** By definition, kyphosis is an exaggerated outward curve of the spine; lordosis is an exaggerated inward curve of the spine (more commonly seen in the cervical and lumbar sections of the spine).

11. **D** Remember LIPS—Latissimus dorsi, the action of Internal rotation, Pectoralis major, and Subscapularis. These muscles are the internal rotators of the shoulder.

12. **A** Bending at the waist not only puts pressure on the back, but it also probably means too much pressure is being exerted on an extended wrist which can lead to wrist/hand problems.

13. **C** The anterior cruciate ligament is one of two ligaments situated behind the patella that connects the femur to the tibia.

14. **A** Visceral muscle needs to be smooth in order for organ functions to occur such as digestion.

15. **B** The vastus lateralis is one of the four quadriceps muscles. All four muscles insert at the tibial tuberosity.

16. **A** Golgi tendons protect the muscle from over-contracting; muscles spindles protect the muscle from over-stretching; the stretch reflex is the combined action of the two that occurs when stretching properly. Proprioceptors assist us with balance and movement in relation to space.

17. **C** The infraglenoid fossa is in the shoulder (scapula); the pubis symphysis is in the anterior middle of the pelvis. The ischium is the bottom portion of the pelvis (ischial tuberosity, that on which we sit).

18. **C** The lateral malleolus is the distal end of the fibula. Distal means farthest away; proximal means closest to.

19. **A** Mastication is chewing.

20. **B** The six hip rotators are gemellus superior, gemellus inferior, obturator internus, obturator externus, piriformis, and the quadratus femoris.

21. **C** The vastus lateralis does not cross the pelvis; it only crosses the knee joint, and the os coxae is on the pelvis.

22. **A** The pectoralis major originates on the clavicle and ribs 1 through 6; the brachialis originates on the shaft of the humerus.

23. **A** While the tibialis anterior inserts on the base of the first metatarsal, it dorsiflexes the foot. Remember muscles pull; they don't push.

24. **A** Comminuted is shattered; compression is fractured by a compressive force; and compound is a fracture that breaks through the skin.

25. **A** These joints are also the synovial joints (the moveable ones).

26. **B** The deltoid ligament is in the ankle, the glenoid labrum is in the shoulder, and the femoral-acetabulum is in the hip joint.

27. **A** Third degree means tearing has occurred—a complete tear. This would also possibly tear the joint capsule causing synovial fluid to spread throughout the joint. Blood vessels would also possibly be torn which would cause the bleeding and bruising.

28. **D** The sciatic nerve runs through or under the piriformis, so tightness of this muscle can cause pressure on the nerve and mimic sciatica.

29. **A** Rectus femoris and vastus lateralis are a part of the quadriceps group which extends, or straightens, the knee. Gluteus maximus extends the hip.

30. **B** SITS = Supraspinatus, Infraspinatus, Teres minor, Subscapularis.

31. **A** The deltoid tuberosity is the insertion of the deltoid muscle.

32. **A** The pectoral nerve innervates the pectoral muscles; the long thoracic muscles innervate the thoracic region. There is no trapezius nerve.

33. **A** The infraglenoid tubercle is the origin of the long head of the triceps, the question asked for the insertion. The other two choices are attachments for biceps brachii.

34. **D** One muscle not included is biceps brachii.

35. **A** Brachialis, biceps, and brachioradialis flex the elbow; supinator supinates the forearm, pronator teres pronates the forearm, and oracobrachialis flexes the shoulder.

36. **B** This is the elbow area (anterior side).

37. **C** This refers to the top of the head (scalp).

38. **D** The acetabulum is also referred to as the hip joint.

39. **B** Movement of the tibia anteriorly or posteriorly are handled by the ACL and the PCL. There is no such ligament in the knee as the inferior or superior cruciate. The patellar ligament attaches the patella to the tibial tuberosity and is commonly lumped in with the patellar tendon.

40. **A** The shoulder is the most mobile as a ball and socket joint but also the most injured.

41. **C** Inversion would be tibialis anterior.

42. **D** The temporomandibular joint is a hinge joint.

43. **B** This is the basic definition of paresthesia—the prickly, burning, tingling feeling you get in a limb when a nerve is damaged or compressed; also, it is the same feeling you get when your arm falls asleep.

44. **D** Hinge, ball and socket, condylar, saddle, pivot, gliding are all synovial joints.

45. **D** Cuneiform is one of the tarsals. The other carpal bones are the pisiform, triquetrum, capitate, trapezoid, and trapezium.

46. **C** Biceps femoris is one of the hamstring muscles; the others are part of the quad group.

47. **D** The medial and longitudinal arches place the pressure points on heads of metatarsals one and five and the heel (calcaneus).

48. **C** Latissimus dorsi does not border the neck.

49. **C** The other choices could be ball and socket joints or condyloid (abduction/adduction or medial/lateral rotation). Hinge joints move like a door on a hinge.

50. **B** Periosteum is the fascia around bones. Fibrocartilage cushions between bones.

51. **A** Syndemosis is a type of fibrous joint but not a class.

52. **C** This is also known as the dens.

53. **A** This is the movement as if you are nodding "yes."

54. **C** This is the movement as if you are nodding "no."

55. **C** The others are cartilage; thymus is a gland.

56. **D** Gracilis is located on the medial thigh and does not border the popliteal fossa (which is the area behind the knee joint).

57. **C** Epicondyle and tuberosity are more for muscle attachments, not articulation. A fossa is not a rounded bump but a rounded groove such as the olecranon fossa of the humerus.

58. **B** The nerve located at this point of the leg is the tibial nerve.

59. **D** The femoral triangle is in this area which includes the femoral artery and nerve.

60. **B** When internal heat goes up, blood vessels dilate in order for blood flow to reach the superficial areas, thus causing us to sweat. This requires an increase in pulse and an increase in metabolism.

61. **A** Ellipsoidal joints allow for flexion, extension, abduction, and adduction. Rotation is not permitted.

62. **D** An inversion ankle sprain means the sole of the foot has turned inward. That means the muscles on the lateral side have been stretched and need to be strengthened.

63. **B** This is also an endangerment site where the carotid artery is located (also where we often take a pulse).

64. **D** Ligaments are slow to heal because they receive little or no blood supply.

65. **B** Both C and D are made-up terms.

66. **D** The word "iliac" helps with this one.

67. **A** It is both the radius and the ulna that allow for pronation and supination movements at the wrist/hand.

68. **A** The rectus femoris is a part of the quadriceps group.

69. **B** Review bony landmarks; coracoid process is on the scapula.

70. **A** Connective tissue includes fascia, tendons, ligaments, skin, and other material.

71. **D** Scalenes attach to the transverse process of C2–7, trapezius attaches to C1–T12, and the splenius capitus attaches to C7–T3. SCM attaches to the medial clavicle and sternum and inserts on the mastoid process.

72. **B** Because of the attachments of the three scalenes on ribs one and two, and along with the pec minor attachments on ribs three through five, tightness in this area can compress these blood vessels.

73. **D** Exchange of gases is the respiratory system.

74. **A** Just like it sounds, the word itself reveals the location.

75. **C** Although the shoulder can be pretty complicated, it's not the largest. The hip is the largest joint.

76. **B** Muscle spindles are stretch sensitive only, baroreceptors are pressure sensitive, and proprioceptors are balance sensitive.

77. **C** Review muscle anatomy: gastrocnemius crosses the knee joint (originates on the femoral condyles) and the ankle joint (attaches to the calcaneus).

78. **B** Ligaments attach bone to bone and therefore work to create a stabilized joint.

79. **D** The sciatic nerve runs either through or just under the piriformis (it can be either). Therefore, if it is tight, the nerve will be compressed and will create sciatica symptoms.

80. **D** Circumduction is flexion, abduction, extension, and adduction, and the abduction/adduction does not occur at this joint. Gliding occurs at the carpal joints.

81. **A** The problem here is when he or she lies down his or her back arches and is unsupported. That would mean an anterior pelvic tilt and tightness in the quadratus lumborum, rectus femoris (quad), and iliopsoas. The best answer choice, then, is "A". Quadratus femoris is a hip rotator, and biceps femoris is a hamstring and if tight, would posteriorly tilt the pelvis.

82. **C** The serratus anterior helps keep the scapula flat along the rib cage when they are retracted.

If the muscle is weak, the scapula stick out or look like wings

83. **B** In other words, the semitendonosis sits on top of the semimembranosis.

84. **D** Water soluble and fat soluble are vitamin classifications.

85. **C** The other bones are not sesamoid bones.

86. **B** Answer "A" is wrong because the diaphragm is not used in forced expiration.

87. **B** Review bony landmarks: shoulder separation is a third degree sprain of the AC ligament (or the sternoclavicular ligament which is not listed here).

88. **B** Because of the effect on the blood vessels (vascular), it can affect vision, balance, and other senses which is why migraines can be so terrible.

89. **B** It is also found in between the tibia and femur (also called meniscus) and between the pubic bones. Hyaline cartilage is on the ends of moveable bones.

90. **A** Skull and C1 moves flexion/extension.

91. **C** The appendicular skeleton includes the appendages (arms, legs, hands, feet); as far as axis goes, there is an axis vertebrae and atlas but not an axis skeleton system. Diarthrotic skeleton is a made-up term.

92. **B** Say Grace before Tea—Sartorius, Gracilis, semi-Tendonosis.

93. **B** Remember *General Manager*: Golfer's elbow is *Medial* epicondyle.

94. **B** Atlas holds up the world (Greek mythology), so the atlas holds up the head.

95. **D** Remember that parasympathetic has the "parachute" (the "para") that slows us down; therefore, the vigorous massage will stimulate the sympathetic system.

96. **C** Proprioceptors are more for balance; nociceptors are for detecting pain.

97. **A** This allows clotting to occur.

98. **D** That would be nerve tissue.

99. **A** These are your moving joints, and synovial fluid helps to lubricate them.

100. **C** Meissner's corpusles detect light pressure; Pacinian's detects pressure and respond to skin displacement and high frequency vibration; Krause's end bulbs are believed to respond to cold. Free nerve endings are the pain receptors.

101. **D** The endomysium encloses each muscle fiber. The perimysium is a fascial layer within the muscle that binds the fasciculi together. The ectomysium does not exist.

102. **C** The five categories are long, short, flat, irregular, and sesmoid.

103. **B** Strokes such as petrissage with the pulling and tugging can activate the muscle spindles for protection of overstretching.

104. **D** Fibrocartilage and meniscus are the same and are found between bones; hyaline cartilage is around the ends of bones.

105. **B** Saturated and unsaturated pertain to fats; water or fat soluble to vitamins.

106. **D** Blood, cartilage, tendons, ligaments are all connective tissues.

107. **C** Another name for adipose tissue is fat tissue. Fat doesn't move.

108. **B** This is what allows us to move.

109. **B** The joint capsule holds the connective tissue and synovial fluid together to nourish the joints but is not considered a main type of connective tissue in the skeletal system.

110. **D** The medial and lateral condyles of the tiba are insertions.

111. **B** Cervical (7), thoracic (12), lumbar (5), sacrum (5 fused). Remember, breakfast at 7, lunch at 12, dinner at 5.

112. **D** Zygomatic is the cheekbone; masseter is the jaw muscle; mandible is the lower jaw bone.

113. **A** The nociceptors detect pain, photoreceptors are related to vision, and chemoreceptors detect taste and smell.

114. **D** These are the muscles in between the metacarpals and the metatarsals.

115. **B** Marrow is the soft material in the bone containing blood cells and other material. The other terms are made up.

116. **D** The capitulum is on the lateral side of the humerus near the lateral epicondyle. The trochlea is closest to the medial epicondyle.

117. **C** The true ribs that articulate with the sternum (hence their name) are ribs one through seven. The false ribs are eight through twelve, and the floating ribs are eleven and twelve.

118. **B** We have more rotation in the neck than anywhere else in the spine (ninety degrees each direction).

119. **C** Remember the mnemonic device: Sally Left The Party (scaphoid, lunate, triquetrum, pisaform) is the proximal row. To Take Cathy Home (trapezium, trapezoid, capitte, hamate) is the distal row.

120. **C** Tibialis anterior performs inversion and dorsiflexion.

121. **D** Because of the TFL/ITB attachment on the anterior crest of the ilium, it can tilt the pelvis anteriorly if tight.

122. **C** Biceps femoris is the hamstring group. If you remember that the rectus abdominus is on the anterior side of the body, it might help you to remember that the rectus femoris is on the anterior side—quads!

123. **B** Quads and abs are muscle groups not individual muscles. The gluteus maximus is the strongest; the sartorius is the longest.

124. **C** Muscle tone is a state of continuous, partial contraction, so the muscles stay systemically stimulated. It allows us to stay upright. Atrophy is the decrease in size of a muscle. The sliding filament theory explains how a muscle contracts via the myosin and actin.

125. **C** Heat stroke occurs when the thermoregulatory system has shut down. Body temperature can rise to very dangerous levels and cause permanent brain damage and even death.

126. **A** By definition, kyphosis is an exaggerated outward curve of the spine, and lordosis is an exaggerated inward curve of the spine (more commonly seen in the cervical and lumbar sections of the spine).

127. **A** Think of the Great Plains of the Midwest: they are flat, so are feet that have pes "planus."

128. **C** The pancreas and stomach are on the left side.

129. **A** This will help to lengthen the low back and put the client in a more neutral pelvic position which would be more comfortable. Remember, lordosis is sway back.

130. **A** Passive stretching means the therapist does the work, and/or both antagonistic and agonistic muscles are relaxed. Active means the client does the work and/or the antagonistic muscle is contracting to stretch the agonist.

131. **A** The "S" in synergist and the "S" in same: the synergist performs the same movement as the primary mover (agonist).

132. **D** Normal daily activities should not create repetitive stress injuries.

133. **B** If the hamstrings are the antagonist, the quadriceps are the agonist. The quads perform knee extension and hip flexion (rectus femoris).

134. **D** The bicep only acts on the shoulder joint, not the girdle (meaning the scapula and clavicle). The other muscles either act on the scapula or attach to the clavicle and therefore are girdle muscles.

135. **B** This is mainly due to the true rib attachments.

136. **B** The supraspinatus initiates abduction, then, at about seventy to eighty degrees, the medial deltoid takes over. Latissiumus dorsi performs adduction, and the subscapularis performs external shoulder rotation.

137. **D** The peroneals attach to the base of metatarsals and therefore do not affect the development of plantar fasciitis directly. Old shoes will lower shock absorption, high arches will tighten the fascia, and low arches will stretch it.

138. **B** Because of gravity, the quadriceps are doing the work to make sure the body doesn't slam down into the chair. Even though the knees are flexing and hamstrings do that, gravity must be taken into account.

139. **B** The gluteus medius and minimus abduct the hip. Gluteus max extends the hip, gracilis adducts the hip, and hamstrings extend the hip.

140. **C** The temporalis is on the skull by the ears; the ethmoid bone is part of the nasal/sinus cavity and forms part of the orbital wall. The pterygoid provide attachments of muscles for the lower jaw and soft palate.

141. **B** The gracilis is on the medial thigh, and the iliotibial band is on the lateral thigh.

142. **D** The masseter originates on the lower border of the zygomatic arch and inserts on the mandible. Remember, muscles pull, they don't push, it makes sense that it closes the jaw.

143. **A** The masseter closes the jaw, the orbicularis oris is the "kissing" muscle (helps us pucker!), and the temporalis muscle elevates and retracts the mandible.

144. **B** Another term for scapular protraction is scapular abduction.

145. **C** Scalenes elevate the first and second rib; the pectoralis minor elevate the ribs. The external intercostals also elevate the ribs.

146. **B** The quadratus lumborum originates on the inferior surface of rib twelve and the transverse processes of the lumbar vertebrae. It inserts on the iliac crest. When the muscle pulls or tightens, it lifts the hip upward.

147. **A** The trapezius sits on top of the rhomboids; therefore, the correct term is superficial.

148. **C** When lying prone, our feet tend to be extremely plantar flexed, or pointed.

149. **B** The metacarpals are further away from the midline than the carpals, and the terms distal and proximal are used for the upper extremities.

150. **C** Sartorius performs hip flexion, external rotation, and knee flexion.

151. **B** This would be an anterior pelvic tilt which would mean the hip flexor muscles would be tight (quads, iliopsoas), and the hip extensors would be stretched and weakened.

152. **C** Eastern anatomical position is with the arms overhead, palms facing forward. The other terms do not exist.

153. **D** The movement described is internal rotation. Remember LIPS for Latissimus dorsi, the action of Internal rotation, Pectoralis major, and Subscapularis.

154. **C** Not only is it due to the lateral malleolus being lower than the medial, but the deltoid ligament on the medial side of the ankle is also very strong. Both of these help prevent more eversion ankle sprains.

155. **A** Because the muscles are contracting, but there is no joint movement (you are stuck halfway up), everything is in an isometric contraction.

156. **C** The medial collateral and lateral collateral ligaments prevent rotation of the knee. The anterior and posterior cruciate ligaments prevent forward or backward motion of the femur on the tibia.

157. **A** The supraspinatus initiates shoulder abduction.

158. **B** The origin is the immoveable end, and the insertion is the moveable end. Ligaments attach bone to bone and have no direct involvement with muscle movement.

159. **C** The bucinnator compresses the cheeks, the masseter is a chewing muscle, and the platysma is the sheath on the anterior neck.

160. **D** There is no iliacus major.

161. **D** This would affect the lumbar spine the most and cause an exaggerated inward curve of the spine.

162. **B** Supraspinatus initiates humeral abduction.

163. **C** Drop foot means the client is unable to dorsiflexes the foot. The muscle that doriflexes is anterior tibialis.

164. **A** Biceps femoris is a part of the hamstrings group. Concentrically, it extends the hip and flexes the knee.

165. **D** The biceps brachii performs shoulder flexion and elbow flexion.

166. **C** Because of gravity, the erector spinae controls trunk flexion in an eccentric way when standing or sitting, which is why we don't work our abs from this position.

167. **A** Anterior tibialis performs dorsiflexion; therefore, walking only on the heels will strength it.

168. **A** Retraction is pulling the mandible backward. Closing the jaw is elevation; opening the jaw is depression.

169. **A** Remember LIPS—Latissimus dorsi, Internal rotation, Pectoralis major, and Subscapularis.

170. **D** Amino acids are proteins; lipids and triglycerides are fats. Meats generally fall into the protein category.

171. **B** Pronation is a combination of dorsiflexion and eversion, and supination is a combination of plantar flexion and inversion.

172. **A** The semitendonosis and semimembranosis attach medial tibia. The rectus femoris, being a part of the quadriceps group, inserts on the tibia, but extends the knee.

173. **A** Hip flexion is what needs to occur, so it would not be the hamstrings since they are involved in hip extension. The vastus lateralis and medialis do not cross the hip joint and therefore do not perform hip flexion.

174. **C** Cervical lamina is an area of the neck, not a muscle.

175. **B** Because gravity is acting downward on the body, the quads are lengthening and contracting in order to prevent you from falling.

176. **D** Remember I Like Spaghetti: ILS are the first letters of each muscle.

177. **B** Distal means farthest away which would be the phalanges. The tarsals are more proximal, and the carpals are in the hands.

178. **C** Remember adduction means you're "adding" everything towards the midline (or spine), so when you retract something, you take it back; therefore, the scapula are pulling back towards the spine.

179. **B** Stabilizers prevent motion; therefore, the rectus abdominus (along with the erector spinae) would be a stabilizer in order to prevent trunk flexion. The gastroc/soleus is an assister because the foot goes from dorsiflexion into slight plantar flexion, movement is taking place there. Hamstrings are antagonist; quads and gluteus max are the primary movers. Iliopsoas at the hip is an antagonist because the hip is extending (but not hamstrings because the knee is extending, and that is quads!).

180. **C** Vitamin A is a fat soluble vitamin, meaning the body cannot expel overdoses easily; it gets stored in the fat. B and C overdoses are excreted through the urine because these vitamins are water soluble.

181. **B** There are six basic nutrients: water, fat, protein, carbohydrates, vitamins, and minerals.

182. **A** Herbs should be treated as medicine; many of them are used as such. You wouldn't ask friends about dosages for prescription medicine or increase your prescription dosages if they don't work immediately, so you do not want to do that with herbs.

183. **D** While many herbs are wonderful for many situations, garlic has been shown to be an excellent antibiotic.

184. **B** Protein recommendations are twelve to twenty percent, fats less than thirty percent, and unsaturated fats ten to twenty percent.

185. **C** HDL and LDL are types of cholesterol. The "S" in Saturated, and the "S" in Sorry: saturated fats are the sorry fats.

186. **B** High glycemic foods have to do with the glucose which is a simple sugar. Since carbs are the primary fuel source, after exercise it is better to eat the high glycemic foods to replace the energy burned for fuel. Mid-to-low glycemic is better before exercise, so a rush of sugar does not enter the bloodstream and cause a spike in energy.

187. **C** Vitamins and minerals both are a basic nutrient with no calories, but minerals are the ones needed in small, trace amounts.

188. **A** A, D, E, and K are fat soluble vitamins. Water soluble vitamins (B and C) will be excreted in the urine if taken in large amounts, but the fat soluble will not.

189. **C** One gram of protein or carbohydrates equals four calories; one gram of fat equals nine calories.

190. **D** The purpose of the glucose is for energy. Too little or too much produces an undesirable effect. While five to ten percent is acceptable, six to eight percent is ideal.

191. **D** Fortified milk has vitamin D.

192. **B** Potassium can be easily flushed out of the body with diuretics, and thus causes cramping. Some doctors will advise or prescribe a potassium supplement in severe cases or recommend eating bananas or potato skins (plain!).

193. **D** Creatine and chromium are both involved in the Kreb's cycle which produces ATP (chemical energy). Although potassium is a mineral, it is a component in muscle contractions but does not assist in the production of ATP.

194. **A** Aloe vera has an antiseptic cooling effect which is wonderful for minor burns.

195. **A** Too much sugar can actually suppress the immune system.

Pathology

chapter 3

CHAPTER OUTLINE

AREAS OF COMPETENCE

This chapter includes sections that correspond to the organization of the NCBTMB exam as follows:

NCETM (14%)

A. Medical terminology
B. Etiology of disease

C. Modes of contagious disease transmission (e.g., blood, saliva)

D. Signs and symptoms of disease

E. Psychological and emotional states (e.g., depression, anxiety, grief)

F. Effects of life stages (e.g., childhood, adolescence, geriatric)

G. Effects of physical and emotional abuse and trauma

H. Factors that aggravate or alleviate disease (e.g., biological, psychological, environmental)

I. Physiological healing process

J. Indications and contraindications/cautions

K. Principles of acute versus chronic conditions

L. Stages/aspects of serious/terminal illness (e.g., cancer, AIDS)

M. Basic pharmacology

- Prescription medications
- Recreational drugs (e.g., tobacco, alcohol)
- Herbs
- Natural supplements

N. Approaches used by other health professionals

NCETMB (12%)

Same as above with the following additions:

O. Approaches used in Western medicine by other health professionals

P. Approaches used in Eastern medicine by other health professionals

Strategies to Success

Study Skills

Remember the SQ3R study system.

Survey the books and chapters that you will use for studying; Re-word the chapter headings as *Questions*; *Read* your book and make notes; *Recite* the material out loud—especially if you are an auditory learner. This helps to burn it in your brain. *Review* right after reading and the next day. In fact review at least every other day to retain the information in your memory.

Pathology is the study of disease, focusing on how the disease changes the function and structure of tissues and organs. As massage therapists and bodyworkers, we know that contraindications—which means no treatment until cleared by a physician—may be due to the disease itself but sometimes is due to the treatment (such as with chemotherapy). In order to provide the best care and treatment plan possible for our clients, we must understand pathology and treatment and follow protocol on who to treat and how to treat them.

Acute: The acute stage of injury or infection is short term (usually a few days or a few weeks). Typically, acute conditions have a sudden onset and run a severe course. Examples include a cold, a sprained ankle, or poison ivy.

Chronic: The chronic stage of injury or infection is either low intensity or long term and in some cases lasts a lifetime. Examples include osteoarthritis, osteoporosis, diabetes, or emphysema.

Disease: Disease is any deviation or interruption of the normal structure or function or a part or organ of the body. The pathology or prognosis may be known or unknown.

Etiology: Etiology is the study of the factors that cause disease and how they come into contact with the human body.

Morbidity: Morbidity is the condition of being sick.

Mortality: Mortality is the death rate of a disease.

Pathophysiology: Pathophysiology is the study of physiology of disease, in other words, how the disease itself functions, grows, and reproduces.

- *endemic*: is when an infectious disease is present in a geographical area or population.
- *epidemic*: is when an infectious disease appears in a new population that spreads at an unexpected, alarming rate.
- *pandemic*: is when an infectious disease spreads world-wide.

Medical Terminology

Before we progress into diseases, it is helpful to review basic medical terminology. This terminology helps us to understand and break down words, some of which may be unfamiliar. See Table 3-1 for basic terminology for the massage therapist and bodyworker.

TABLE 3-1

At a Glance: Medical Terminology

Root/ Prefix/Suffix	Meaning	Example
A-, an-	Without	Anesthesia
Acetabul-	Vinegar, cup	Acetabulum
Ad-	Toward	Adduct
Adip-	Fat	Adipose
Agglutin-	To glue together	Agglutination
-algia	Pain	Myalgia
Aliment-	Food	Alimentary canal
Alveoli-	Small cavity	Alveoli
Ambi-	Both	Ambidextrous
An-	Without	Anaerobic
Ana-	Build up	Anabolic
Angio-	Vessel	Angioplasty
Ante-	Before	Antebrachium
Anti-	Against	Antibiotic
Append-	To hang something	Appendix
Arthro-	Joint	Arthritis
Bi-	Two	Bicep
-blast	Budding	Osteoblast
Brachio-	Arm	Brachioradialis
Brady-	Slow	Bradycardia
Bronch-	Windpipe	Bronchiole
Cardio-	Heart	Cardiology
Cata-	Break down	Catalyst
Caud-	Tail	Caudal
Cephal-	Head	Cephalad
Chondro-	Cartilage	Chondromalacia
-clast	Broken	Osteoclast
Cochlea	Shell	Cochlea

TABLE 3-1 CONTINUED

Root/ Prefix/Suffix	Meaning	Example
Con-	Together	Contract
Condyl-	Knob	Femoral condyle
Contra-	Against	Contraindicated
Cort-	Covering	Cortex
Cyano-	Blue	Cyanotic
Cyt-	Cell	Cytoplasm
Derm-	Skin	Dermatologist
Di-	Two	Diarthrotic
Diastole-	Dilation	Diastolic blood pressure
Diuret-	To pass urine	Diuretic
Dors-	Back	Dorsal
Dur-	Tough	Dura mater
Dys-	Hard, painful, difficult	Dyspnea
Ecto-	Outside	Ectopic pregnancy
-ectomy	Surgical removal	Appendectomy
Ede-	Swelling	Edema
Embol-	Stopper	Embolus
Endo-	Within	Endoplasmic reticulum
Epi-	Upon	Epidermis
Ergo-	Work	Ergonomics
Erythr-	Red	Erythrocyte
Ex-, exo-	Outside	Excrete
Extra-	Outside	Extracellular
Folic-	Small bag	Hair follicle
For-	Opening	Foramen
Gangli-	A swelling	Ganglion cyst
Gastro-	Stomach, belly	Gastrointestinal
-genic	Produce, create	Pathogenic
Glen-	Joint socket	Glenoid fossa
Glosso-	Tongue	Glossopharyngeal
Glycol-	Sugar	Glycolosis
Hemi-	Half	Hemisphere
Hemo-, hema-	Blood	Hemophylia
Hepa-	Liver	Hepatitis
Histo-	Tissue	Histology
Homeo-	Same	Homeostasis

At a Glance: Medical Terminology

Root/Prefix/Suffix	Meaning	Example
Hydro-	Water	Hydroculator
Hyper-	Above	Hypertrophy
Hypo-	Below	Hypotonic
-iatric	Specialty	Pediatrics
Ilio(a)-	Ileum	Iliac crest
Infra-	Below	Infraspinatus
Inter-	Between	Interphalangeal
Intra-	Inside	Intracellular
-ism	Condition	Hyperthyroidism
Iso-	Same	Isometric
-itis	Inflammation	Arthritis
Kine-	Movement	Kinesiology
Later-	Side	Lateral
Leuko-	White	Leukocyte
Lipo-	Fat	Liposuction
Lyso-	Break up	Lysosome
Macro-	Big	Macrophage
Mal-	Bad	Malpractice
Mater	Mother	Dura mater
Medi-	Middle	Medial
Melan-	Black	Melanoma
Multi-	Many	Multifidus
Myo-	Muscle	Myofibril
Nephron-	Kidney	Nephritis
Neuro-	Nerve	Neurology
Odont-	Tooth	Odontoid process
-ology	Study of	Kinesiology
-oma	Tumor	Neuroma
Ora-	Mouth	Oral
Ortho-	Straight	Orthopaedist
Osteo-	Bone	Osteoarthritis
Oto-	Ear	Otoscope
Para-	Beside, near	Paraspinals
Patho-	Disease	Pathology
-penia	Lack of	Osteopenia

TABLE 3-1 CONTINUED

Root/Prefix/Suffix	Meaning	Example
Peri-	Around	Periosteum
-plegia	Paralysis	Paraplegic
Pneumo-	Breathing	Pneumonia
Pod-, ped-	Foot	Pedal
-poiesis	Formation	Hemopoiesis
Poly-	Many, much	Polymyalgia
Pre-	Before	Premature
Quadri-	Four	Quadriceps
Rect-	Straighten	Rectus abdominus
Reno-	Kidney	Renal disease
Sclero-	Hardening	Scleroderma
-sis	Process	Stenosis
Somato-	Body	Somatic healing
Steno-	Narrowing	Stenosis
Sub-	Under, below	Subscapularis
Super-, supra-	Above	Supraspinatus
Syn-	Together	Synapse
Systole-	Contraction	Systolic blood pressure
Tachy-	Fast	Tachycardia
Tetan-	Stiff	Tetanus
Thermo-	Heat	Hyperthermia
Thoraco-	Chest	Thoracic vertebrae
Thrombo-	Clot	Thrombosis
Trans-	Across, over	Tranverse process
Tri-	Three	Tricep brachii
-tomy	Cutting	Anatomy
-trophy	Growth	Hypertrophy
Uni-	One	Unilateral
-uria, -uro	Urine	Dysuria
Vaso-	Vessel	Vasoconstriction
Ventr-	Belly or stomach	Ventricle of the heart
Viscero-	Organ	Viscerotropic

The Nine Regions of the Abdomen

There are nine abdominal regions in the body (Figure 3-1). Medical professionals refer to these regions when describing structures or abnormalities/diseases, especially since our vital organs are located here.

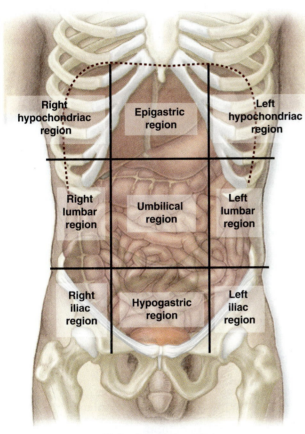

Right hypochondriac region
Epigastric region
Left hypochondriac region
Right lumbar region
Umbilical region
Left lumbar region
Right iliac region
Hypogastric region
Left iliac region

Abdominopelvic regions

Figure 3-1 The nine abdominal regions.

Risk Factors for Disease

The following are conditions that put us at a higher risk for developing disease. Some of these risk factors can be prevented while others cannot.

Age: As we get older, our bodies get older. Exercising and proper nutrition may slow this process, but certain conditions will still occur. For example, our arteries will not be as elastic and will begin to harden, possibly leading to high blood pressure. This in turn can lead to a lesser ability to transport oxygen efficiently, which may in turn affect the health of tissue. Our muscular tissue loses elasticity as well, causing muscles to lose some flexibility. Muscle mass also begins to decline which in turn can affect metabolism. In women especially, hormonal changes affect many aspects of health, placing women at higher risk for heart attacks.

Gender: Some diseases are related to gender. These can include prostate cancer, ovarian cancer, breast cancer, and immune conditions.

Genetics: Genes play a role in the occurrence of some diseases such as cancers and possibly heart disease. This is due to an actual defect in the gene that has been passed down from a previous generation.

Physical exposure: Some jobs and environments can increase our risk of certain diseases. For example, skin cancer is caused by too much sun exposure. Emphysema may arise from work conditions involving fumes, particles, and pollutants if the proper respiratory equipment or gear is not used or available.

Nutrition: Poor nutrition can lead to conditions such as cancers and diabetes. Eating foods high in hydrogenated fats can cause the LDL (bad) cholesterol to increase and the HDL (good) cholesterol to decrease, thus increasing one's risk of heart attacks.

Congenital defects: Congenital defects include conditions or diseases present at birth, such as heart defects. For example, a young athlete who collapses and dies is later found to have a heart defect that was unknown or undetected.

Occupational hazards: Examples of occupational hazards include repetitive stress syndrome such as carpal tunnel, stress on the job, and physical exposures.

Pre-existing conditions: This is different from congenital defects in that these may have formed after birth, for example, an old football injury in high school that led to arthritis of the knee.

Lifestyle and habits: Lifestyle and habit risk factors can include choices that keep you from or put you at risk for injury, accidents, or disease, for example, using your seat belt, using sunscreen, or drinking adequate water.

Microorganisms

Microorganisms are tiny microscopic living things that can have an impact on our health. They fall into several categories, but the ones that are most relevant to our health are noted below.

Bacteria: Bacteria are primitive one-celled organisms. Some bacteria are harmless and actually benefit our health, such as acidophilus (which helps to control the bad bacteria in our digestive system). Examples of bacterial infections include strep throat, gonorrhea, acne, and bacterial meningitis. The typical medical treatment for a bacterial infection is antibiotics. See Table 3-2.

Fungi: Fungi are one-celled plants that are responsible for breaking down organic matter in the environment. Yeast is a form of fungi. The yeast that infects the body is called *Candida albicans*. Other fungal infections include athlete's foot, nail rot, and ringworm. See Table 3-3.

Protozoans: Protozoans are one-celled animals that have a cell that includes organelles. An example of a protozoan is the amoeba. Most amoebas are harmless;

TABLE 3-2

At a Glance: Etiology of Disease—Bacteria

Organism/Pathogen	Reservoir	Infection/Disease
Escherichia coli	Colon, manure	Food poisoning, diarrhea, enteritis
Staphylococcus aureus	Skin, hair, nose	Cellulites, pneumonia, impetigo, acne, boil
Streptococcus pneumoniae	Throat, skin, lungs	Pneumonia
Streptococcus pyogenes	Throat, skin	Strep throat, scarlet fever, rheumatic fever
Mycobacterium tuberculosis	Lungs	Tuberculosis
Neisseria gonorrhoeae	Genitalia, rectum, mouth	Gonorrhea
Borrelia burgdorferi	Tick	Lyme disease
Clostridium botulinum	Food (improperly handled)	Botulism, food poisoning, gastroenteritis
Salmonella enterididis	Food (improperly handled)	Salmonella, food poisoning, gastroenteritis
Helicobacter pylori	Duodenum, stomach, saliva	Ulcers

TABLE 3-3

At a Glance: Etiology of Disease—Fungi

Organism/Pathogen	Reservoir	Infection/Disease
Candida albicans	Mouth, skin, genitalia, intestines	Candidiasis, thrush, dermatitis
Epidermophyton floccosum	Skin	Athlete's foot, ringworm, jock itch

however, some can cause a deadly diseases such as dysentery. See Table 3-4.

Viruses: In order for a virus to survive because it is so primitive, it must enter another living cell or "host." Having entered the body, it uses the cell organelles (ribosomes, mitochondria, nucleus, etc.) to make copies of itself. Examples of virus infections are influenza, polio, HIV, measles, and viral meningitis. Since viruses have no cellular metabolism of their own, they cannot be neutralized with antibiotics. See Table 3-5.

TABLE 3-4

At a Glance: Etiology of Disease—Protozoa

Organism/Pathogen	Reservoir	Infection/Disease
Plasmodium falciparum	Mosquito	Malaria
Trichomonas vaginalis	Urinogenital tract	Trichomoniasis
Entamoeba histolytica	Water, food, feces	Amoebic dysentery

TABLE 3-5

At a Glance: Etiology of Disease—Viral

Organism/Pathogen	Reservoir	Infection/Disease
Human immunodeficiency virus	Body fluids	AIDS
Influenzavirus type A, B, C	Droplets, lung	Influenza
Paramyxovirus	Droplets	Measles, mumps, respiratory infections
Human papillomavirus	Skin	Warts
Herpes virus types 1 and 2	Mucous membrane, genitalia, rectum, blisters	Herpes simplex, genital herpes

Modes of Disease Transmission

Two things that can help lower the risk of contacting some diseases is practicing healthy habits and being careful. As massage therapists and bodyworkers, one of the easiest ways for us to reduce our risk is by washing our hands. This will help lessen disease transmission via direct physical contact (actually touching the client or the diseased area). Direct physical contact can occur in three ways.

1. **Mucous membranes**: Pathogens can enter through mucous membranes. This can be as simple as touching a contaminated area on a client and then rubbing your eye; you have possibly transmitted the pathogen into your eye membranes.
2. **Intact skin**: This can occur with fleas, scabies, lice, ticks, fungi, poison oak or ivy, or through an insect bite or sting.
3. **Broken skin**: This allows the pathogen to enter through a break in the skin. For example, a bite from an animal, surgery, skin eruptions, hangnail, or IV access can allow bacteria to enter the open area or even into the blood stream through an open blood vessel.

Indirect physical contact is another method of disease transmission. Indirect physical contact means the infected person does not need to touch someone directly to pass the disease. We see this often during cold and flu season with sneezing and coughing. There are two methods of indirect contact.

1. **Ingestion**: This can be via contaminated water, undercooked meats, or foods not properly handled, stored, or refrigerated. *E. coli* and dysentery are transmitted this way.
2. **Inhalation**: Pathogens can be inhaled or absorbed through the respiratory mucosa by coming in contact with airborne droplets or body fluids (e.g., blood, saliva) through coughing or sneezing. Tuberculosis is transmitted this way.

Signs of Inflammation

Inflammation is the body's protective mechanism to stabilize an area, to contain an infection, and to begin the repair process. The extent of the inflammation is directly proportional to the degree of trauma. This is important to massage therapists and bodyworkers because it means an acute situation is going on within the client's body. Massage therapists and bodyworkers want to avoid treatments in the case of inflammation in order to allow the body to heal. The stages of inflammation are explained below.

Redness: This is the first stage of the inflammation process. It occurs because the blood vessels dilate to allow white blood cells to travel to the trauma site. Remember, white blood cells help our bodies rid themselves of bacteria and other pathogens. The vasodilation allows for the white blood cells to permeate the capillary walls

Swelling: The vasodilation of the capillary walls allows blood plasma to merge into the interstitial spaces which causes the increased swelling.

Heat: The heat occurs because of the vasodilation.

Pain: As pressure in the tissue increases, it places stress and stimulation on the nerve receptors resulting in pain. This pain can lead to muscle splinting, thus causing more pain and a limit in the range of motion of related joints.

This leads to the pain cycle (Figure 3-2). The pain cycle can be due to inflammation as described above or any kind of painful stimulus that results in a muscle contraction with muscle splinting or guarding. When we have muscle movement, waste products form. If the muscles continue to move, the blood vessels dilate, enabling the waste products to be extracted from the muscles and removed from the body. If guarding or splinting occurs, we not only constrict the blood vessels, but we also prevent the waste products from being removed. These waste products (such as lactic acid) can

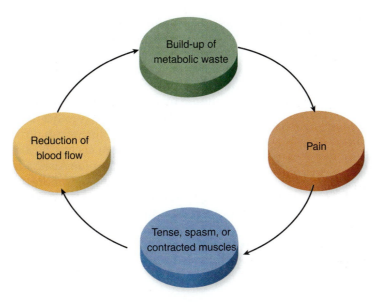

Figure 3-2 The pain cycle.

build up and cause more swelling. The swelling creates more pain and more restricted movement, and the cycle repeats itself. Massage helps to break this cycle by relaxing the splinted muscles, thus dilating the blood vessels and manipulating the removal of the waste products and excess interstitial fluids.

Disorders / Diseases

Now that we understand diseases and injuries better, let's look at specific diseases and how they relate to treatment options for massage and bodywork. First, we need to discuss a few terms.

Medical clearance: Medical clearance is a form or letter from a physician stating that the doctor's patient (your client) can receive a massage without any restrictions, can receive a massage but with restrictions, or cannot receive a massage based on the information you—the

therapist—have provided the doctor. Remember, the doctor cannot divulge information about his/her patient to you since this would violate patient/doctor confidentiality. You must also receive authorization from your client to discuss this with the physician. The legality of this will be discussed in Chapter 6.

Indicated: "Indicated" means that a massage or bodywork can be given to a client without a clearance from a doctor. Generally this means your client does not have any conditions or health issues that warrant restrictions or clearances from his/her physician.

Indicated with restriction: This means your client has a condition that warrants a modification to the massage but does not necessarily warrant a medical clearance from the doctor. For example, the client may have osteoporosis. You can still massage this client, but you must adjust your pressure to accommodate for the brittle bones and the risk of fracture and damage with deep pressure. Or you may have a client with an undiagnosed

Memory Helper
When in doubt, refer it out.

but serious shoulder injury. In this case, you could avoid the injured shoulder but massage elsewhere. Remember, we are not doctors and cannot diagnose. See Table 3-6.

Absolute contraindications: This means that the massage cannot be given until further notice from the client's physician. Keep in mind, this does not necessarily mean the client needs to actually see his/her doctor. If he/she has seen their doctor within the past six months to a year, the physician will most likely let you know without seeing them again. Sometimes it is not the disease itself that is the concern but the course of treatment, such as chemotherapy. Other times it's not the disease itself but the other problems that come with it, such as AIDS. (Remember, people don't die of AIDS, they die of opportunistic conditions due to their suppressed immune systems.) We need to make sure our clients are stabilized enough to receive massages that are beneficial and not harmful. We as practitioners *Do No Harm.* Another example would be diabetes. Because this disease can be life-threatening, we need to make sure our client's glucose is stabilized and that no other complications are occurring such as neuropathy, arteriosclerosis, and more. Who better to ask than the doctor because sometimes the patient doesn't know, has forgotten, or, sadly, isn't concerned. See Table 3-6.

TABLE 3-6

At a Glance: Diseases or Disorders That Are Indicated With Restrictions

Acne	
Boils	
Bunions	(avoid vigorous massage over bunion area)
Burns	
Bursitis	(do not massage over affected area if acute)
Cerebral palsy	(if sensation is present, massage is indicated)
Contractures	(if sensation is present)
Edema	(if not acute and only due to soft tissue injury)
Epilepsy	(except during seizures)
Fibromyalgia	(care must be taken not to overtreat)
Gallstones	(if symptom free and no draining strokes over the liver/gallbladder area)
Gout	(in non-acute stage, avoid gouty joints at all times)
Hematoma	(local contraindication in acute phase; light, gentle massage in chronic phase)
Hernia	
Herniated disc	(massage is indicated in subacute phase)
Impetigo	(lesions need to heal before any massage is given)
Irritable bowel syndrome	(avoid abdominal area)
Multiple sclerosis	(contraindicated in acute flare-up; is indicated in subacute phase, but avoid deep tissue and heat therapies)
Osteoarthritis	(locally contraindicated in acute flare-ups, otherwise OK to massage)
Osteoporosis	(use light pressure so as not to damage bones further)
Psoriasis	(local contraindication in acute stage)
Rheumatoid arthritis	(contraindicated during acute flare-ups)
Tendonitis	(local contraindication)
Varicose veins	(local contraindication and distal to the varicose veins)

TABLE 3-6 CONTINUED

Disorders/Diseases with *Absolute Contraindications* for Massage (Do not massage at all and refer to doctor, or massage with doctor's supervision)

Alcoholism	
Alzheimer's disease	
Amyotrophic lateral sclerosis	(Lou Gehrig's disease)
Anemia	(if advanced pernicious, hemolytic, aplastic, and secondary anemias)
Aneurysm	
Ankylosing spondylitis	
Atherosclerosis	(especially if advanced)
Bronchitis	(especially if contagious)
Cancers	(most and depending on where they are with treatment)
Cirrhosis	(if advanced)
Congestive heart failure	
COPD/emphysema	
Crohn's disease	(massage under medical supervision, avoid abdominal area)
Diabetes	
Diverticulitis	(in the presence of active infection, otherwise avoid the abdominal area)
Edema	(caused by systemic problems such as congestive heart failure)
Emphysema	
Fever	
Gout	(in acute phase)
Hemophilia	
Hepatitis	
HIV/AIDS	(due to other diseases caused by AIDS)
Hypertension	(need to rule out underlying cause)
Leukemia	
Lupus	(if in acute flare-up, may be indicated in subacute phase per doctor)
Impetigo	
MI or angina pectoris	
Osteomalacia	
Parkinson's	
Pleurisy	
Scleroderma	(need to make sure skin is healthy and sensation is normal, must see doctor)
Seizures	
Shingles	
Stroke	
Substance abuse	(should be under doctor's care if client is currently recovering)
Thyroid disease	(underlying cause needs to be found)

Occasionally our clients have signs or symptoms but have not seen a physician. When we interview our clients to discuss how they are feeling, these signs and symptoms may be brought to our attention. See Table 3-7. Massage therapists and bodyworkers should be familiar with these so that we can refer them to a doctor (and make note of it in our documentation which will be discussed in Chapter 6). Some of these signs and symptoms may warrant a contraindication for massage which also must be noted in our documentation. Again remember, we do not diagnose, we evaluate.

TABLE 3-7

At a Glance: Signs and Symptoms of Disease

Disease	Signs/Symptoms	Massage Implications
Alcoholism—dependency on alcohol.	Symptoms are increased tolerance to the effects of alcohol, memory loss (blackouts), neglect in other responsibilities.	Massage is appropriate if the person is recovering from alcohol abuse under medical supervision. Contraindicated if they are currently under the influence.
Alzheimer's disease—progressive degeneration of the brain leading to dementia.	Many signs exist, but the most common are memory loss, delusions, personality changes, and social withdrawal.	Since massage is not likely to cause harm, it can be indicated with a medical clearance and within the comfort level of the client.
Ankylosing spondylitis—a progressive arthritis of the spine.	First signs are usually stiffness and pain around the sacrum. Advanced stages cause the client to be locked in a flexed position.	A medical clearance is needed; however, massage is contraindicated in acute flare-ups.
Asthma—spasmodic constriction of the bronchial tubes with excess mucous production.	Symptoms are coughing, wheezing, and difficulty breathing, especially while exhaling.	Massage is indicated unless the client is having an attack. The client should keep his/her inhaler with him/her during the massage.
Atherosclerosis—arteries become occluded due to plaque.	Generally, there are no symptoms until it becomes advanced. However, other problems can increase the risk, such as circulatory problems, hypertension, coronary artery disease, and diabetes.	Massage is contraindicated for advanced artherosclerosis. Medical clearance is advised if they know they have it or have one of the other diseases listed as related.
Bronchitis—inflammation of the trachea, bronchi, and bronchioles, either acute or chronic (chronic can be caused by smoking, exposure to chemicals, or other environmentally unsafe inhalants).	Symptoms for acute include infection, fever, fatigue, difficulty in breathing, coughing, and wheezing. Symptoms for chronic include difficulty breathing, coughing, and constant wheezing.	Massage is contraindicated for acute bronchitis. Medical clearance is needed for chronic bronchitis because of other related diseases such as emphysema and lung cancer.
Bursitis—inflammation of the fluid-filled sac (bursa). Bursas protect muscle and tendon from rubbing over bone during movement.	Symptoms are pain with movement in the affected area.	Massage is indicated with restriction; generally, massage can be given, but the bursitis area should be avoided.

TABLE 3-7 CONTINUED

Disease	Signs/Symptoms	Massage Implications
Cancer—the growth of malignant cells.	Early signs depend on the area of the body affected.	Although benefits exists in giving massage to someone with cancer, because of treatments for the cancer, medical clearance is necessary, especially on the timing of massage when receiving chemotherapy in order to maximize the therapy without flushing it out of the system too quickly.
Chronic fatigue syndrome— a group of symptoms that indicate a stressed immune system.	Symptoms are debilitating fatigue, possibly accompanied by fever, muscle aches, headaches, and swollen lymph nodes.	Massage is indicated and very beneficial
Cirrhosis—when normal liver cells are replaced with scar tissue.	Early symptoms include loss of appetite, nausea, vomiting, and weight loss. Advanced symptoms include jaundice and vomiting blood.	Massage is contraindicated in advanced cirrhosis. Medical clearance is necessary for all other cases.
COPD/Emphysema—where the alveoli sacs in the lungs are dying off.	Symptoms are shortness of breath with mild exertion and cyanosis (bluish lips and fingernails).	Medical clearance is needed.
Crohn's disease—inflammatory disease of the small intestines and sometimes large intestines.	Symptoms are diarrhea, abdominal pain, and weight loss.	Massage is indicated with restriction, with no abdominal massage. Medical clearance for general massage is suggested, however.
Dermatitis/Eczema—inflammation of the skin. Eczema is a non-contagious skin rash.	Dermatitis can manifest as large wheals, such as from poison ivy, or less inflammation. Eczema usually looks like very dry, flaky skin.	For dermatitis, it depends on the cause. If it is from poison ivy and could spread, massage is contraindicated. If the skin is very inflamed, blistered, or red, it is indicated with restriction with avoidance of the inflamed area.
Diabetes Mellitus—elevated glucose or glucose intolerance.	Symptoms are frequent urination, thirst, increased appetite with weight loss (especially Type I). Type II symptoms are being overweight and increased triglycerides with increasing glucose levels.	Medical clearance is suggested to ensure that tissues are healthy and diabetes is under control.
Diverticulosis/Diverticulitis— development of small pouches in the colon that can become inflamed and/ or infected.	Diverticulosis usually lacks symptoms; however, when inflamed (diverticulitis), one can experience lower left-side abdominal pain, cramping, bloating, constipation, or diarrhea.	If infection is present, massage is contraindicated. If there is no infection but the client has diverticulosis, massage is indicated with restriction, which is no abdominal massage.
Edema—the retention of interstitial fluid. Causes can vary.	Tissue is puffy. If there is a local infection, it may be warm to the touch.	Massage is contraindicated for most edema, especially if the cause is unknown. If it is due to an acute injury such as an ankle sprain, massage is indicated with restrictions, which would be to avoid the area in a general massage.

TABLE 3-7 CONTINUED

At a Glance: Signs and Symptoms of Disease

Disease	Signs/Symptoms	Massage Implications
Embolism/Thrombus— thrombi are stationary clots; emboli are clots that travel.	If it lodges in an organ, such as the heart, it can cause tissue death (heart attack) or brain death (stroke).	Massage is <u>contraindicated</u>.
Epilepsy—seizure disorder.	Symptoms are seizures. However, the type of seizure will vary from person to person.	Massage is <u>indicated</u> unless a current seizure is occurring.
Fibromyalgia—chronic muscle pain, trigger points, and non-restorative sleep.	Fibromyalgia is diagnosed through process of elimination and eleven of eighteen trigger points are positive and widespread.	Massage is <u>indicated</u>.
Glomerulonephritis—glomeruli (small structures within the nephrons) are inflamed or do not function.	Symptoms are dark or rust colored urine, foamy urine, or blood in urine.	Massage is <u>contraindicated</u>.
Gout—inflammatory arthritis caused by deposits of uric acid.	This usually affects the big toe but not always. Affected joints become hot, red, swollen, and extremely painful.	In the acute phase, massage is <u>contraindicated</u>. Other times, massage is <u>indicated with restrictions</u> with avoidance of the affected joints.
Heart attack (myocardial infarction)—damage to the heart muscle due to lack of oxygen, possibly due to plaque.	Symptoms are angina, shortness of breath, chest pressure, and possible pain around the jaw, left arm, and back (especially in women).	<u>Medical clearance</u> is required prior to a massage after recovery from a heart attack to ensure stabilization.
Hematoma—a deep bruise with leakage of blood between the muscle sheaths.	Symptoms are pain, sometimes with a visible bruise if superficial. A bump that feels fluid-filled can oftentimes be felt.	Massage is <u>indicated with restrictions</u>, not massaging over or around the hematoma.
Hepatitis—inflammation of the liver, usually due to a virus.	Symptoms are fatigue, jaundice, abdominal pain, nausea, and/or diarrhea. Sometimes, however, no symptoms exist until the latter stages.	Massage is <u>contraindicated</u> in the acute phase and requires medical clearance in the chronic phases.
Herniated disc—bulging disc possibly putting pressure on the associated spinal nerve.	Symptoms are referred pain along the dermatome, muscle weakness, and/or paresthesia.	Massage is <u>indicated with restrictions</u> in the acute phase in which the area is avoided. Massage is indicated in the chronic phase.
HIV/AIDS—Acquired Immune Deficiency Syndrome caused by the human immunodeficiency virus (HIV).	Symptoms are weakness or flu-like symptoms, but often no symptoms appear in the early stages.	<u>Medical clearance</u> is necessary prior to massage to ensure other underlying problems do not contradict the massage.

TABLE 3-7 CONTINUED

Disease	Signs/Symptoms	Massage Implications
Hypertension—elevated blood pressure with the systolic at 140 or higher, OR the diastolic at 90 or higher. Must be diagnosed by physician.	There are no definitive symptoms, which is why it is called "the silent killer."	For moderate or borderline high blood pressure (HBP), massage can be <u>indicated</u> to help reduce stress; however, <u>medical clearance</u> is appropriate. For HBP that requires medication, <u>medical clearance</u> is needed since underlying cause may contradict the massage.
Hyperthyroidism—too much thyroid hormone is available.	Symptoms are unexplained weight loss, intolerance to heat, nervousness, insomnia, and palpitations.	<u>Medical clearance</u> is needed to confirm the underlying cause is found and is under control.
Hypothyroidism—too little thyroid hormone is available.	Symptoms are weakness, fatigue, unexplained weight gain, intolerance to cold, hair loss, and brittle nails.	<u>Medical clearance</u> is needed to confirm the underlying cause is found and is under control.
Impetigo—bacterial infection of the skin.	Symptoms are a rash with fluid-filled blisters and honey-colored crust. Usually begins on the face.	Massage is <u>contraindicated</u> because this is a staph infection and is affecting the client systemically. It is also very contagious.
Irritable bowel syndrome—spasms and other dysfunctions of the digestive system.	Symptoms alternate between diarrhea and constipation, bloating or abdominal distention, and abdominal cramps relieved with bowel movements.	Massage is <u>indicated with restrictions</u>, which are to avoid abdominal massage.
Lupus—autoimmune disease in which connective tissue is attacked by antibodies.	Symptom is a characteristic butterfly rash. Generally, lupus clients also have arthritis in two or more joints and kidney/nervous system dysfunction.	Massage is <u>contraindicated</u> during acute flare-ups because it is systemic. Medical clearance is needed for massage in the chronic state.
Multiple sclerosis—destruction of the myelin sheaths around motor and sensory neurons.	Many symptoms exist including fatigue, eye pain or twitching, loss of hearing in one ear, and clumsiness.	Massage is <u>contraindicated</u> during flare-ups because it is systemic. It is <u>indicated</u> if there is no flare-up; however, deep tissue and heat (such as hot packs, paraffin baths) should be avoided.
Osteoarthritis—joint inflammation due to wear and tear of the bone.	Symptoms are stiffness and pain usually affecting weight-bearing joints.	Massage is <u>indicated with restriction</u> during acute flare-ups by avoiding the inflamed joint but otherwise indicated.
Osteoporosis—loss of bone mass.	This is diagnosed by X-ray. In later stages, symptoms would be easily fractured bones.	Massage is <u>indicated with restrictions</u>, which are to use lighter pressure.
Parkinson's disease—degenerative disease of cells of the brain that produce dopamine.	Early signs include resting tremor of hands, feet, or head, stiffness, and poor balance. Dopamine helps basal ganglia to maintain balance, posture, and coordination, so these are affected.	<u>Medical clearance</u> is needed prior to massaging these clients.

TABLE 3-7 CONTINUED

At a Glance: Signs and Symptoms of Disease

Disease	Signs/Symptoms	Massage Implications
Psoriasis—a non-contagious skin disease.	This occurs in pink or reddish patches that sometimes look scaly.	Massage is <u>indicated with restriction</u> with avoidance of open sores.
Renal failure—the kidneys are not functioning. It can be acute or chronic but life-threatening either way.	Symptoms vary, but reduced urine output, systemic edema, and changes in mental state because of toxicity are common.	Massage is <u>contraindicated</u> for both acute and chronic.
Rheumatoid arthritis—auto-immune disease where the synovial membranes are attacked by the immune system.	In acute phase, joints become red, swollen, and warm to the touch. Joints often become misshapen.	Massage is <u>contraindicated</u> in acute flare-ups because the flare-up is systemic. If there is no flare-up, massage is <u>indicated</u>.
Stroke—damage to the brain by either a clot or an aneurysm.	Symptoms are paralysis, slurred speech, numbness on one side, sudden extreme headache.	<u>Medical clearance</u> is needed prior to massage.
Tendonitis—inflammation of a tendon usually due to overuse.	Pain and stiffness with movement.	Massage is <u>indicated with restriction</u> with avoidance of the inflamed area in the acute phase and indicated in the chronic phase.
Thrombophlebitis or deep vein thrombosis	Symptoms are inflammations of veins due to blood clots.	Massage is <u>contraindicated</u>.
Ulcers—Sores that remain open for various reasons. Gastric ulcers are more common.	With gastric ulcers, burning abdominal pain usually occurs between meals.	Massage is <u>indicated with restriction</u> with no abdominal massage.
Varicose veins—blood pooling in the veins usually of the lower extremities due to valve damage within the vein.	Symptoms are ropey, slightly bluish veins usually found in the lower legs.	Massage is <u>indicated with restrictions</u> with no massage around the vein and distal to them.
Warts—caused by extremely slow acting viruses.	These look cauliflower shaped and are usually found on hands.	Massage is <u>indicated with restriction</u> which is avoidance of the wart area because it is contagious.

Massage and Cancer

Cancer has always been a controversial area for massage therapists and bodyworkers. However, it is important to understand the stages of cancer in order to better understand the treatment procedure taken. Treatment options vary and depend on the stage of cancer, type of cancer, and the choice made between patient and doctor. Table 3-8 provides a description of the various stages of cancer. Always remember to check with your client's physician before proceeding with massage. Treatment options can affect the frequency and timing of the massage. For example, massage immediately following chemotherapy might flush the chemicals out of the client's body too quickly; therefore waiting twenty-four to seventy-two hours after the treatment might be best. The client's physician can help in this decision.

TABLE 3-8

At a Glance: Stages of Cancer	
Stage One	This consists of a small lump which has invaded the tissue beyond the lobules or ducts, but it has not yet spread to lymph nodes or the other parts of the body.
Stage Two	There is a slightly larger tumor size, or there are enlarged lymph nodes which indicate more trouble may be imminent. There is no sign of distant metastases for stage two either.
Stage Three	The cancer is larger than two inches in diameter, or it has invaded other areas or surrounding skin. Lymph nodes are enlarged. Tests of the liver, lungs, and bones show no concrete cancer on these organs.
Stage Four	The cancer is detectable in other organs.

Drugs and Herbal Therapy

We have discussed medical conditions that might warrant a contraindication to a massage, but sometimes other conditions or situations apply. While the "inappropriate client" will be discussed in Chapter 6, there is another type of client you may encounter: the client under the influence of drugs or alcohol. Below are effects of various recreational drugs to alert us to the possibility that a massage should not be given.

Recreational drugs: These are drugs that are not required for a medical condition but wanted because of how they make the user feel. They are generally, but not always, illegal. The drug itself can cause injury, complications, and even death. Because massage can heighten the affect of these drugs, massage is contraindicated if there is suspicion of use. See Table 3-9.

Prescription Drugs: Prescription drugs are prescribed by a physician for a particular problem, health issue, or disease. They can only be dispensed by a pharmacy and cannot be purchased over the counter. Massage may have an undesirable affect because of the medication or vice versa. For example, many arthritis medications can cause an ulcer. This would prevent the therapist from performing abdominal massage and would therefore be considered a condition that is indicated with restriction. See Table 3-10.

TABLE 3-9

At a Glance: Recreational Drugs and Effects

Drug	Classification	Effect
Alcohol	Depressant	Dizziness, slurred speech, disturbed sleep, impaired motor skills, violent behavior, death in high doses
Amphetamines "Speed"	Stimulant	Anxiety, increased blood pressure, aggression, violent behavior, dilated pupils, progressive deterioration with heavy use
Methamphetamines "Meth, crank"	Stimulant	Anxiety, increased blood pressure, paranoia, stroke, depression, convulsions, toxicity, hallucinations
Ecstasy	Stimulant	Panic, anxiety, depressions, paranoia, muscle tension, tachycardia, HBP, drug craving, hallucinations
Cocaine	Stimulant	Pupil dilation, elevated vital signs, paranoia, seizures, heart attack, respiratory failure, hallucinations, erratic behavior, death from overdose
Heroin	Opiate	Intense euphoria, slowed and slurred speech, constricted pupils, droopy eyelids, impaired night vision, respiratory depression or failure, dry skin, skin infections
Inhalants (vapors, aerosols)	Volatile substances	Intoxication similar to alcohol, muscle weakness, abdominal pain, severe mood swings, violent behavior, nosebleeds, liver/lung/kidney damage, toxicity
Marijuana	Cannabinoid	Bloodshot eyes, dry mouth and throat, altered sense of time, reduced ability to perform tasks requiring concentration and coordination, impaired learning/memory/thinking
Steroids	Steroidal	Mood swings, acne, cardiovascular disease, kidney/liver damage, aggression, sterility, masculine traits in women, feminine traits in men

TABLE 3-10

At a Glance: Prescription Drugs

Condition/Drug	Use	Side Effects
Arthritis (Celebrex, Motrin, Naprosyn)	Anti-inflammatory, arthritic symptoms	GI upset, ulcers, changes in liver enzymes
Blood Pressure		
1. Beta blockers (Lopressor, Tenormin, Atenolol, Propanolol)	Lower blood pressure, also used to treat migraines (especially Inderal)	Hypotension, decreased heart rate, dizziness, GI upset
2. ACE inhibitors	Lower blood pressure (common choice for diabetics with HBP because of lesser effect on glycemic control)	Hypotension, lethargy, GI symptoms
3. Calcium channel blockers (Verapamil, Diltiazem)	Lower blood pressure	Hypotension, dizziness, headache
4. Diuretics	Lower blood pressure by reducing blood volume by causing an increased production of urine	Loss of potassium, muscle cramping
Cancer		
1. Chemotherapy drugs	Used to inhibit the growth of more cancer cells	Nausea, vomiting, hair loss, anemia, immune suppression
2. Tamoxifen (nolvadex)	Used to treat breast cancer	Reduces platelet count, may cause menopausal symptoms such as hot flashes, night sweats, insomnia
Cardiovascular		
1. Antianginals (nitroglycerin)	Lessen chest pain, dilate coronary arteries	Lightheadedness, headache
2. Anticoagulants (Coumadin)	Prevent formation of clots	Bruise easily, tissue or organ hemorrhage, rash, abdominal pain, headache
3. Antihyperlipidemics (Lipitor, Zocor, Questran)	Reduce cholesterol, especially LDLs	GI upset, muscle aches, headache, dizziness, elevated liver enzymes
Diabetes		
1. Insulin	Replace the insulin that the pancreas is unable to produce (as in Type I diabetes)	Hypoglycemia if too much is taken, diabetic coma if too little is taken
2. Glucophage	Stimulates the pancreas to produce more insulin (as in Type II diabetes)	Same as insulin
Hormone Replacement		
1. Androgens	Used to increase testosterone levels	Urinary urgency, breast tenderness
2. Estrogen	Used to treat menopause	Nausea, headaches, edema of lower extremities

TABLE 3-10 CONTINUED

At a Glance: Prescription Drugs

Condition/Drug	Use	Side Effects
Infection		
1. Antibiotic (penicillin, tetracycline, amoxicillin, Cipro)	Destroy or inhibit the growth of bacteria	Nausea, GI upset
2. Antivirals (Zovirax, Retrovir, Symmetrel)	Inhibit viral growth	GI upset, headache, dizziness, insomnia
Thyroid		
1. Hypothyroid meds (synthroid, levithroid)	Treats low thyroid production	Insomnia, irregular heartbeat, shortness of breath, nervousness, heat intolerance
2. Antithyroid meds	Inhibits the production of thyroid for those who have hyperthyroidism	Abnormal components of the blood
Respiratory Conditions		
1. Decongestants	Shrink nasal mucous membranes	Constricts blood vessels, hypertension, irritation to the sinuses (if in a spray)
2. Expectorants	Increase respiratory secretions	Excitability, constipation, nausea, drowsiness
3. Bronchodilators	Relieve bronchospasms, asthmatic symptoms	Hyperactivity, tremors, nervousness, insomnia, tachycardia

Whether it is stress or a medical issue, many often turn to herbs for help. Many think that because herbs are natural, they are harmless. However, herbs, just like prescription drugs, have side effects and contraindications. Table 3-11 presents basic herbs and the pathology for which they may be used. Table 3-12 discusses herbs that should not be used during pregnancy due to risk to the baby, premature contractions, bleeding, or other pregnancy risks. Keep in mind that referral from the appropriate healthcare professional is necessary for recommendation of herbs. This is not in the scope of practice for massage therapists and is only presented here for the purpose of the national exam.

TABLE 3-11

At a Glance: Herbs for Various Pathologies

Pathology	Herb(s)
Acne	Evening Primrose Oil, Raspberry Leaf, Nettle, Dandelion, Lemon Grass
Anemia	Red Beet, Yellow Dock, Lobelia, Burdock, Nettle, Mullein
Colds	Chamomile, Slippery Elm, Cayenne, Goldenseal, Myrrh, Peppermint, Sage, Garlic
Constipation	Aloe Vera, Slippery Elm, Barberry
Coughs	Wild Cherry Bark, Licorice, Comfrey Root
Earaches	Oil of Mullein, Garlic Oil
Flu	Ginger, Cayenne, Goldenseal, Licorice
Heartburn	Fennel Seed, Peppermint, Cinnamon, Lavender
Insomnia	Valerian, Scullcap, Hops
Menopause	Black Cohosh, Licorice, Ginseng, Blessed Thistle
Migraines	Fenugreek, Thyme, Feverfew
Sore throat	Marshmallow, Fenugreek

TABLE 3-12

At a Glance: Herbs to Avoid or Use With Caution During Pregnancy

Angelica	Licorice Root
Black Cohosh	Motherwort
Blue Cohosh	Mugwort
Borage oil	Nutmeg
Comfrey	Pennyroyal Leaf
Dong Quai	Rue
Elder	Saffron
Fenugreek	Shepherd's Purse
Goldenseal	Uva Ursi
Henbane	Yarrow
Horsetail	

Effects of Physical and Emotional Abuse and Trauma

While some clients may have medical issues, others may have emotional or physical abuse or trauma issues. Regardless of its source, an emotional trauma contains three common elements:

- it was unexpected;
- the person was unprepared; and
- there was nothing the person could do to prevent it from happening.

One way to tell the difference between stress and emotional trauma is by looking at the outcome: how much residual effect an upsetting event is having on our lives, relationships, and overall.

Stress: Stress can be good or bad. For example, a vacation can be stressful because of the planning and packing, but it can also be exciting and fun. The body, however, will react in the same way: by vasoconstriction, an increase in blood pressure, and an increase in the sympathetic nervous system. We have stress in our lives every day, but generally are able to control it.

Traumatic distress can be distinguished from routine stress by assessing the following:

- how quickly upset is triggered
- how frequently upset is triggered
- how intensely threatening the source of upset is
- how long upset lasts
- how long it takes to calm down

There are common effects or conditions that may occur following a traumatic event. Sometimes these responses can be delayed for months or even years after the event. Often, people do not even initially associate their symptoms with the precipitating trauma. The following are symptoms that may result from a more **commonplace, unresolved trauma**, especially if there were earlier, overwhelming life experiences:

Physical Symptoms of Trauma

- Eating disturbances (more or less than usual)
- Sleep disturbances (more or less than usual)
- Sexual dysfunction
- Low energy
- Chronic, unexplained pain

Emotional Symptoms of Trauma

- Depression, spontaneous crying, despair and hopelessness
- Anxiety
- Panic attacks
- Fearfulness
- Compulsive and obsessive behaviors
- Feeling out of control
- Irritability, anger, and resentment
- Emotional numbness
- Withdrawal from normal routine and relationships

Cognitive Symptoms of Trauma

- Memory lapses, especially about the trauma
- Difficulty making decisions
- Decreased ability to concentrate
- Feeling distracted

Extreme symptoms can also occur as a delayed reaction to the traumatic event.

Re-experiencing the Trauma

- Intrusive thoughts
- Flashbacks or nightmares
- Sudden floods of emotions or images related to the traumatic event

Emotional Numbing and Avoidance

- Amnesia
- Avoidance of situations that resemble the initial event
- Detachment
- Depression
- Guilt feelings
- Grief reactions
- An altered sense of time

Increased Arousal

- Hyper-vigilance, jumpiness, an extreme sense of being "on guard"
- Overreactions, including sudden unprovoked anger
- General anxiety
- Insomnia
- Obsessions with death

Common Personal and Behavioral Effects of Emotional Trauma

- Substance abuse
- Compulsive behavior patterns
- Self-destructive and impulsive behavior
- Uncontrollable reactive thoughts
- Inability to make healthy professional or lifestyle choices
- Dissociative symptoms ("splitting off" parts of the self)
- Feelings of ineffectiveness, shame, despair, hopelessness
- Feeling permanently damaged
- A loss of previously sustained beliefs

Common Effects of Emotional Trauma on Interpersonal Relationships

- Inability to maintain close relationships or choose appropriate friends and mates
- Sexual problems
- Hostility
- Arguments with family members, employers, or co-workers
- Social withdrawal
- Feeling constantly threatened

*Some questions are not directly addressed in this chapter, but are meant to act as a general review of subjects studied in various school curriculums.

Questions

Pathology
NCETM (14%) NCETMB (12%)

1. When the bronchial tubes become inflamed, constricted, and have an unusual build-up of mucous, this is called
   A. adhesions.
   B. asthma.
   C. atopic lungitis.
   D. tracheotomy.

2. Bursitis can be caused by
   A. overuse.
   B. bacterial infection.
   C. misalignment of joints.
   D. All of the above are correct.

3. Possible underlying causes of edema might include
   A. congestive heart failure.
   B kidney dysfunction.
   C. nutritional deficiencies.
   D. All of the above are correct.
   E. None of the above are correct.

4. The disorder where the bones become brittle and porous is called
   A. osteoarthritis.
   B. scleroderma.
   C. osteoporosis.
   D. osteodermitis.

5. In the age group of twenty-five- to thirty-year-olds, the most common cause of death by disease is
   A. osteoporosis.
   B. squamous dermatitis.
   C. psoriasis.
   D. melanoma.

6. The "ABCDs" of what to look for in a mole include all of the following except
   A. asymmetrical.
   B. big.
   C. color.
   D. diameter.

7. Which of the following conditions is contraindicated for massage?
   A. skin pallor
   B. senile lentigo
   C. psoriasis
   D. impetigo

8. What factor(s) can increase one's risk of having a hip replacement?
   A. lack of treatment
   B. delay in treatment
   C. Both A and B are correct.
   D. None of the above are correct.

9. Psoriasis
   A. has no known cause.
   B. has no known cure.
   C. benefits from exposure to UV light.
   D. All of the above are correct.

10. The most common fracture with osteoporosis is
    A. compound fracture.
    B. compression fracture.
    C. comminuted fracture.
    D. simple fracture.

11. Scleroderma
    A. affects more men than women.
    B. is an autoimmune disorder.
    C. has only been found to be genetic.
    D. Both A and B are correct.

12. The best time to perform a skin check for moles is
    A. adulthood.
    B. at night before bed.
    C. first thing in the morning.
    D. after a bath or shower.

13. If a client's pancreas is not functioning and is producing no insulin, he or she is said to be
    A. type II diabetic.
    B. anemic.
    C. type I diabetic.
    D. adult onset diabetes.

14. If a diabetic client takes too much insulin and does not eat enough food, the blood sugar will probably
    A. drop too low.
    B. go up too high.
    C. stay in normal range.
    D. None of the above are correct.

15. The two main lymphatic ducts drain into the
    A. inferior and superior vena cavas.
    B. left and right subclavian veins.
    C. left and right atriums.
    D. left and right ventricles.

16. Inflammation of the veins is called
    A. angioplasty.
    B. pericarditis.
    C. phlebitis.
    D. aneurysm.

17. Risk factors for diabetes include all of the following except
    A. high cholesterol.
    B. hypertension.
    C. high HDL cholesterol.
    D. smoking.

18. Signs and symptoms of diabetes may include all of the following except
    A. decreased urination.
    B. dry mouth.
    C. slow healing sores.
    D. sudden weight loss.

19. Hardening of the arteries in the circulatory system is called
    A. arteriosclerosis.
    B. atherosclerosis.

    C. aneurysm.
    D. None of the above are correct.

20. Possible contraindications for massage for a client include all of the following except
    A. controlled blood pressure.
    B. congestive heart failure.
    C. varicose veins.
    D. phlebitis.

21. Risk factors for heart disease include the following except
    A. gender.
    B. family history.
    C. low blood sugar.
    D. age.

22. What disease affects the bones and joints and is considered an immune disorder?
    A. osteoporosis
    B. osteoarthritis
    C. rheumatoid arthritis
    D. fibromyalgia

23. The covering around the central nervous system that can deteriorate in a disease such as multiple sclerosis is called
    A. dendrites.
    B. axons.
    C. myelin sheath.
    D. pia mater.

24. For a massage client with cystic fibrosis, which two massage techniques are most beneficial to help loosen phlegm?
    A. rocking and vibration
    B. tapotement and vibration
    C. cupping and rocking
    D. petrissage and tapotement

25. COPD stands for
    A. congestive obstructive pulmonary disease.
    B. chronic obstructive pulmonary disease.
    C. Crohn's obstructive pyloric disease.
    D. congestive obstructive passing disease.

26. Adhesive capsulitis is also known as
    A. hypermobility.
    B. a third degree sprain.
    C. frozen shoulder.
    D. Osgood-Schlatters disease.

27. A client states that he or she has had angina pectoris. This means he or she has
    A. an atrophied pectoralis major.
    B. a hypertrophied pectoralis minor.
    C. had a heart attack.
    D. had chest pain.

28. Uncontrolled high blood pressure can lead to
    A. cerebrovascular accident.
    B. myocardial infarction.
    C. hypotension.
    D. nephritis.

29. Your client states he or she is on a beta blocker for his or her blood pressure. Your concern for your client is
    A. the blood pressure medication will have no affect on his or her heart rate.
    B. the blood pressure medication does have an affect on his or her heart rate and he or she might feel light-headed after his or her massage.
    C. the medication may cause his or her heart rate to rise during the massage and may make him or her light-headed during the massage.

30. Your client states that he or she has been told by his or her doctor to take an aspirin a day for cardiovascular health. Your concern during the massage is
    A. no concerns exist.
    B. possible bruising from too deep of a massage since aspirin is a blood thinner.
    C. possible clots since aspirin can thicken the blood for better transportation of hemoglobin.
    D. changes in pressure due to the analgesic affect.

31. Which of the following conditions requires physician clearance prior to any massage?
    A. chronic pain
    B. asthma
    C. congestive heart failure
    D. a bruise

32. When it is stated that massage may negate medication, this means that
    A. massage will enhance the affects of the medication.
    B. massage will produce the opposite affect wanted by the medication.

C. massage is beneficial with the medication.
    D. massage will have no effect on the medication.

33. The word used to describe the progression of a disease is called
    A. diagnosis.
    B. prognosis.
    C. pathology.
    D. anomaly.

34. Pain is
    A. subjective in nature.
    B. objective in nature.
    C. factual in nature.
    D. the sign of a major problem.

35. When an illness or injury has become "exacerbated," it means the illness/injury
    A. has gotten better.
    B. is genetic or hereditary.
    C. has gotten worse.
    D. has become chronic.

36. When giving your symptoms to the doctor, you are helping him/her determine
    A. the anomaly.
    B. the diagnosis.
    C. the placebo.
    D. objective information.

37. A client informs you, the therapist, that he has a benign, non-infectious, chronic condition. This may mean that the
    A. client may have cancer.
    B. client may have periods of good days/bad days.
    C. condition is not contagious.
    D. condition will go away soon.

38. The stimulus at which the first noticeable muscle contraction occurs is called the
    A. threshold stimulus.
    B. tone.
    C. reflexive stimulus.
    D. contractional stimulus.

39. Characteristics of the inflammatory response include all of the following except
    A. redness.
    B. swollen.
    C. warm to the touch.
    D. cold to the touch.

40. Emphysema is
    A. when the alveoli sacs begin to die in the lungs, and oxygen is unable to get into blood stream for gas exchange.
    B. reversible.
    C. also known as a CAD.
    D. All of the above are correct.

41. Diseases of the liver include
    A. hepatitis and diverticulitis.
    B. cirrhosis and diverticulitis.
    C. hepatitis and cirrhosis.
    D. liverenteritis and hepatitis.

42. Inflammation of the mucous membrane that surrounds the abdominal cavity is called
    A. peritonitis.
    B. gastroenteritis.
    C. pleurisy.
    D. diverticulitis.

43. Inflammation of the fluid surrounding the lungs is called
    A. peritonitis.
    B. pericarditis.
    C. pleurisy.
    D. diverticulitis.

44. Type I diabetes is characterized by
    A. a pancreas that does not function to produce insulin.
    B. seen in older adults.
    C. is also called non-insulin dependent diabetes mellitus.
    D. Both B and C are correct.

45. Type II diabetes is characterized by
    A. a pancreas that produces insulin, but the body resists it.
    B. high family history incidence.
    C. must be treated with insulin.
    D. Both A and B are correct.

46. Inflammation of the urinary bladder is called
    A. nephritis.
    B. dialysis.
    C. cystitis.
    D. uritis.

47. When someone is allergic to the point that his or her trachea closes up, this is called
    A. asthma.
    B. anaphylactic shock.
    C. tracheitis.
    D. pulmonary embolism.

48. Inflammation of the inner ear is called
    A. otitis media.
    B. Addison's disease.
    C. temporal otitis.
    D. conjunctivitis.

49. Which of the following will NOT predispose someone to disease?
    A. age
    B. nutrition/diet
    C. driving habits
    D. lifestyle

50. Necrosis is
    A. another term for a blood clot.
    B. infection of the nephron.
    C. tissue death.
    D. another term for a pulmonary embolism.

51. When the skin turns yellowish in color due to a buildup in bilirubin, this is called
    A. cyanosis.
    B. jaundice.
    C. conjunctiva.
    D. cystitis.

52. Chest pains with radiation down the left arm and up the jaw are also known as
    A. heart murmur.
    B. embolism.
    C. angina pectoris.
    D. myocardial disease.

53. Orthostatic hypotension is
    A. elevation of the blood pressure in response to an injury.
    B. a drop in the blood pressure from staying in the same position too long.
    C. a condition that is contraindicated for massage.
    D. Both A and C are correct.

54. Torticollis is
    A. forward head position.
    B. a spasm causing lateral flexion of the neck.
    C. a spasm causing extension and flexion/rotation of the neck.
    D. a curvature of the thoracic spine.

55. A condition that has sudden onset and the symptoms last a short amount of time is called
    A. acute.
    B. chronic.
    C. virulent.
    D. minor.

56. When the body produces too much cortisol due to too much adrenocorticotropic hormone, the disease that occurs is called
    A. hyperthyroidism.
    B. Cushing's disease.
    C. diabetes.
    D. hypothyroidism.

57. Another name for myalgia is
    A. multiple sclerosis.
    B. osteoarthritis.
    C. muscle pain.
    D. osteoporosis.

58. Glaucoma is
    A. a detached retina.
    B. inflammation of the lacrimal glands.
    C. a growth that forms in the eye.
    D. increased pressure in the eye.

59. A viral infection related to chicken pox whose pustules follow along a nerve path making it very painful is called
    A. impetigo.
    B. psoriasis.
    C. shingles.
    D. seborrhea.

60. Emphysema is described as
    A. infection of the pleural cavity.
    B. spasms of the bronchiole tubes.
    C. overproduction of phlegm.
    D. destruction of the alveoli sacs.

61. The abnormal deterioration of articular cartilage and joint is called
    A. osteoarthritis.
    B. osteoporosis.
    C. rheumatoid arthritis.
    D. articulitis.

62. What type of disease or illness does NOT respond best to antibiotics?
    A. bacterial infection
    B. urinary tract infection
    C. viral infection
    D. All of the above respond to antibiotics.

63. A pandemic disease is one in which
    A. the community is affected.
    B. a continent is affected.
    C. the entire world is affected.
    D. a state is affected.

64. Virulence means
    A. the ability of an organism to cause a disease.
    B. the ability for a disease to be deadly.
    C. the ability for viruses to be destroyed through medication.
    D. the strength of a virus and its morbidity rate.

65. A disease that hardens the epithelial cells in the skin and digestive tract is called
    A. rheumatoid arthritis.
    B. gout.
    C. scleroderma.
    D. cystitis.

66. Natural passive immunity is
    A. the ability of a mother to pass antibodies to her unborn child.
    B. the ability of the body to absorb nutrients through food.
    C. homeopathic treatment for disease.
    D. None of the above are correct.

67. The purpose and function of histamine is to
    A. cause vasodilatation.
    B. produce of antibodies.
    C. increase the permeability of blood vessels.
    D. Both A and C are correct.

68. Another name for kidney stones is
    A. nephritis.
    B. cystitis.
    C. urolithiasis.
    D. hepatitis.

69. Another name for tinea cruris is
    A. athlete's foot.
    B. jock itch.
    C. plantar warts.
    D. drop foot.

70. The disease that is caused by a decrease in dopamine production and is characterized by impaired motor functions, poor balance, slow speech, and a shuffling gait is called
    A. Bell's palsy.
    B. Alzheimer's disease.
    C. Parkinson's disease.
    D. senility.

71. Another term for pathologically dry skin is
    A. impetigo.
    B. ichthyosis.
    C. psoriasis.
    D. seborrhea.

72. Inflammation of a tendon and/or the surrounding synovial sheath is called
    A. a strain.
    B. tendonitis.
    C. tenosynovitis.
    D. a sprain.

73. An avulsion is
    A. the tearing away of a tendon from its bony attachment.
    B. the tearing away of a ligament from its attachment.
    C. a type of fracture.
    D. None of the above are correct.

74. The absence of menstruation is called
    A. vaginitis.
    B. dysmenorrhea.
    C. amenorrhea.
    D. endometriosis.

75. Pes planus means
    A. high arches in the foot.
    B. low arches in the foot.
    C. normal arches in the foot.
    D. irriation of the plantar fascia.

76. A tumor in the bone tissue is called
    A. osteoma.
    B. myoma.
    C. carcinoma.
    D. lipoma.

77. Scoliosis can be caused by
    A. leg length discrepancy.
    B. carrying a purse on the same shoulder.

    C. postural alignment abnormality.
    D. All of the above are correct.

78. Decubitus ulcers
    A. are pressure sores.
    B. occur only in the cubital area of the arm.
    C. generally occur in short-term bed illness.
    D. are not preventable.

79. Protruding, irregular rope-like veins are called
    A. phlebitis.
    B. venules.
    C. spider veins.
    D. varicose veins.

80. A condition where the vertebral body of one of the lumbar vertebrae is anterior compared to the rest of the spine is called
    A. spondylosis.
    B. spondylolisthesis.
    C. osteoarthritis.
    D. semispinalis.

81. Amyotrophic lateral sclerosis is also known as
    A. scleroderma.
    B. Lou Gehrig's disease.
    C. spondylitis.
    D. multiple sclerosis.

82. A contracture is
    A. an indication for massage.
    B. permanently shortened muscles.
    C. usually found in flexion of the joint.
    D. All of the above are correct.

83. Abdominal massage would be contraindicated for
    A. Crohn's disease.
    B. constipation.
    C. small fibroids.
    D. All of the above are correct.

84. A syndrome where circulation is affected in the extremities that makes the client sensitive to cold is called
    A. Raynaud's syndrome.
    B. pyelonephritis.
    C. peritonitis.
    D. peripheral vascular disease.

85. Thoracic outlet syndrome can be caused by
    A. hypertonic scalenes.
    B. hypotonic pectoralis minor.

C. structural abnormalities in ribs three to five.

D. hypertonic trapezius.

86. A crackling sound heard in joint movements that oftentimes is abnormal is called
    A. cyanosis.
    B. tenosynovitis.
    C. crepitus.
    D. spondylosis.

87. If symptoms are alleviated without curing the underlying disease, it is called
    A. palliative.
    B. palpable.
    C. paresis.
    D. paraplegia.

88. A deficiency of iodine in the diet can lead to
    A. goiter.
    B. diabetes.
    C. low blood pressure.
    D. hypoglycemia.

89. Which group is most prone to osteoporosis?
    A. premenopausal women
    B. postmenopausal women
    C. young girls between the ages of eleven and twenty-four
    D. All of the above are correct.

90. What can cause rickets in children?
    A. lack of calcium
    B. lack of exercise
    C. lack of vitamin D
    D. lack of fluoride in the water

91. When stress goes beyond the body's normal limits, this is called
    A. disease.
    B. strain.
    C. sprain.
    D. anomaly.

92. When the placenta separates prematurely from the uterine wall, it is called
    A. ectopic pregnancy.
    B. abruptio placentae.
    C. preeclampsia.
    D. spontaneous abortion.

93. If a client comes to you with psoriasis and is requesting a massage, what should you do?
    A. Make sure you wash and clean the area before giving the massage
    B. Tell the client politely that you cannot give them a massage because it is contraindicated
    C. Proceed with the massage, but avoid the area
    D. Refer them to a physician for clearance

94. Immunity developed after coming in contact with a disease is called
    A. active artificially acquired immunity.
    B. active naturally acquired immunity.
    C. passive naturally acquired immunity.
    D. vaccination.

95. A partial dislocation is called a
    A. subluxation.
    B. paridislocation.
    C. sprain.
    D. strain.

96. If an elderly client who appears to have kyphosis and low back pain cames to you, your best course of action is to
    A. perform the massage using deep pressure.
    B. seek the doctor's advice because you suspect osteoporosis.
    C. perform a light massage.
    D. focus on relieving the pectoralis major and hip flexors.

97. Muscles that decrease in size are going through
    A. hypertrophy.
    B. myotrophy.
    C. atrophy.
    D. dystrophy.

98. A deficiency in vitamin B12 may result in
    A. pernicious anemia.
    B. rickets.
    C. osteoporosis.
    D. osteomalacia.

99. A fibroid is a/an
    A. benign tumor.
    B. superficial skin tumor.
    C. melanoma.
    D. inflammation of muscular tissue.

100. Another term for hypertension is
    A. stress.
    B. low blood pressure.
    C. high blood pressure.
    D. cerebrovascular accident.

101. Accumulation of the cerebrospinal fluid around the brain it is called
    A. encephalitis.
    B. meningitis.
    C. hydrocephalus.
    D. hyrdrocranialitis.

102. Coarctation of the aorta is a/an
    A. aneurysm.
    B. localized narrowing of the aorta.
    C. localized necrosis of the aorta.
    D. blockage of the aorta.

103. A thrombus is a
    A. stationary blood clot.
    B. moving clot.
    C. hardening of the arteries.
    D. paresthesia.

104. An ulceration in the mucosal lining of the stomach is called
    A. peptic ulcer.
    B. diverticulosis.
    C. fundal ulcer.
    D. reflux.

105. When the thyroid secretes too much hormone leading to weight loss, nervousness, insomnia, etc., this is called
    A. Graves' disease.
    B. hypothyroidism.
    C. Cushing's disease.
    D. diabetes mellitus.

106. A sprain can occur in which structures?
    A. muscle
    B. tendon
    C. bony prominence
    D. ligament

107. The medical field of physical medicine and rehabilitation is called
    A. physiology.
    B. physiatry.

    C. psychology.
    D. psychiatry.

108. The healing of the body by means of manipulation is called
    A. physiotherapy.
    B. hydrotherapy.
    C. mechanotherapy.
    D. psychiatry.

109. Conditions or situations that merit caution and adaptive measures to ensure the massage is safe and that the client is comfortable are called
    A. relative contraindications.
    B. absolute contraindications.
    C. endangerment sites.
    D. indications.

110. Which of the following is not an indication for massage?
    A. stress, anxiety, and insomnia
    B. phlebitis, thrombus, and varicosity
    C. muscle soreness
    D. myofascial pain

111. What term is used to describe an observable reddening of the skin resulting from increased blood flow?
    A. ischemia
    B. hypoxia
    C. anemia
    D. hyperemia

112. Another term for subcutaneous layer is
    A. hypodermis
    B. subdermis
    C. dermis
    D. epidermis

113. Degenerative joint cartilage is found in which disorder?
    A. rheumatoid arthritis
    B. gout
    C. osteoarthritis
    D. bursitis

114. Varicose veins are best described as
    A. localized edema.
    B. knotty appearance under the skin.
    C. purplish under the skin.
    D. little squiggly veins under the skin.

115. Which of the following conditions is most likely to result from stress, poor diet, and lack of exercise?
    A. tendonitis
    B. constipation
    C. migraines
    D. CHF

116. Ankylosing spondylitis generally affects what areas of the body?
    A. immune system
    B. muscles
    C. vertebrae and sacroiliac (SI) joint
    D. all weight-bearing joints

117. The disease where uric acid crystals deposit in a joint causing inflammation is called
    A. gout.
    B. rheumatoid arthritis.
    C. scleroderma.
    D. lupus.

118. Holding one's breath while "bearing down," otherwise known as a Valsalva maneuver, is not a safe thing to do because it
    A. temporarily stops blood flow to the left atrium, then when the maneuver is released, blood floods the atrium.
    B. temporarily stops blood flow to the right atrium, then when the maneuver is released, blood floods the atrium.
    C. increases the risk of blood pooling in the veins and leading to varicose veins.
    D. places undue stress on the intestines.

119. Massaging a large abnormally dilated vein is contraindicated because
    A. a clot can dislodge.
    B. blood would be rushed into the right ventricle causing undue stress on the heart.
    C. the artery would be damaged.
    D. it would flood tissue fluid into the lymph system and slow down the flow of lymph.

120. A condition where the skin is red, scaly, and flakes off is called
    A. eczema.
    B. psoriasis.
    C. impetigo.
    D. scleroderma.

121. The suffix "-itis," as in arthritis, indicates
    A. pain.
    B. inflammation.
    C. damage.
    D. chronic.

122. The type of wart found on the bottom of the foot is called
    A. dorsal.
    B. solar.
    C. plantar.
    D. acute.

123. Your client states that he or she has blood pressure that tends to be on the low side, but no symptoms. You should
    A. not massage him or her.
    B. focus on strokes away from the heart to improve peripheral circulation.
    C. massage him or her as you normally would.
    D. suggest being put on BP medication.

124. A metabolic disorder characterized by excessive thirst and urination and caused by a deficiency in antidiuretic hormone is called
    A. nephritis.
    B. diabetes mellitus.
    C. diabetes insipidus.
    D. edema.

125. Signs and symptoms of emphysema include all of the following except
    A. dyspnea.
    B. fatigue.
    C. loss of appetite.
    D. acute cough.

126. The single greatest risk factor for emphysema is
    A. chemical fumes.
    B. smoking.
    C. heredity.
    D. pollution.

127. Another name for lung cancer is
    A. bronchiogenic carcinoma.
    B. COPD.
    C   pleuralgenic carcinoma.
    D. dyspnocarcinoma.

128. Inflammation of the bladder is called
    A. nephritis.
    B. cystitis.
    C. renalitis.
    D. glomerularitis.

129. Blood in the urine is called
    A. hypoproteinemia.
    B. anemia.
    C. hematuria.
    D. reduced glomerular filtration.

130. Hemiplegia means
    A. total paralysis.
    B. blood disorder.
    C. stroke.
    D. half of vertical body is paralyzed.

131. Risk factors for developing asthma are
    A. low birth weight.
    B. GERD.
    C. family history.
    D. All of the above are correct.

132. Problem(s) associated with asthma are
    A. excess production of mucus.
    B. smaller than normal diameter in the trachea.
    C. fewer alveoli sacs.
    D. Both A and B are correct.

133. GERD stands for
    A. gastroesophogeal reflux disease.
    B. gastroesophogeal reflux disorder.
    C. gastroesophogeal regurgitation disease.
    D. None of the above are correct.

134. Abdominal massage is contraindicated for
    A. Crohn's disease.
    B. colitis.
    C. irritable bowel syndrome.
    D. All of the above are correct.

135. Which of the following would not be a cause for gallstones?
    A. obesity
    B. too little estrogen
    C. ethnicity
    D. cholesterol

136. Which hepatitis virus is not usually chronic?
    A. A
    B. B
    C. C
    D. D

137. A metabolic disorder that is the result of a deficiency in insulin is called
    A. diabetes mellitus.
    B. diabetes insipidus.
    C. gestational diabetes.
    D. Graves' disease.

138. Symptoms of dehydration include
    A. thirst.
    B. increased urination.
    C. moist skin.
    D. All of the above are correct.

139. Another term for varicose veins around the anus is
    A. pruritus ani.
    B. constipation.
    C. hemorrhoids.
    D. fistulae.

140. Diseases that can cause constipation include all of the following except
    A. lupus.
    B. diabetes.
    C. stroke.
    D. All of the above can cause constipation.

141. Which of the following fights bacteria in the body?
    A. platelets
    B. erythrocytes
    C. leukocytes
    D. fibrinogen

142. Why is massage of infections contraindicated?
    A. it isn't
    B. the therapist could get sick
    C. the infection could spread in the client
    D. the germs would linger in the massage room

143. For the client who has phlebitis, which technique should be used?
    A. deep tissue work on the area affected
    B. light tissue work on the area affected
    C. lymphatic drainage
    D. None.

144. What type of massage is beneficial for lupus?
    A. light effleurage
    B. hot packs
    C. tapotement
    D. none

145. Uncontrolled high blood pressure can lead to
    A. cerebrovascular accident.
    B. myocardial infarction.
    C. hypotension.
    D. nephritis.

146. If you are working the left sternocleidomastoid muscle (SCM) and you have the client's head turned to the left, this means the head position is
    A. contralateral.
    B. ipsalateral.
    C. inferior.
    D. proximal.

Answers and Explanations

Pathology
NCETM (14%) NCETMB (12%)

1. **B** These are typical characteristics of asthma. Atopic lungitis is a made-up term. Tracheotomy is when a hole is made in the trachea through the neck in order to attach a hose to a breathing apparatus.

2. **D** All of these can contribute to bursitis.

3. **D** All of the above apply here. If the heart cannot pump blood effectively or the kidneys cannot filter and pass fluid through effectively, then it will build up fluid in the body. Nutritional deficiencies can be due to too much sodium as well as too little protein (kwashiorkor, the distended abdomen commonly seen in Third World countries).

4. **C** Osteoarthritis is wear and tear of the ends of the bones, scleroderma is hardening of the skin and epithelial cells, and osteodermitis is a made-up word.

5. **D** Skin cancer is deadly. The others are not.

6. **B** These are things to look for in a mole that may make it suspicious and need to be looked at by the dermatologist: "A" means asymmetrical (not circular in shape); "B" is border (the border is irregular and not smooth looking); "C" is color (black, orange, red, blue, purple all may be signs of a cancerous mole); and "D" is diameter (a larger-size mole may be cancerous or on the verge of being cancerous).

7. **D** Impetigo is highly contagious through touch while the others are not.

8. **C** A lack of treatment or delay in treatment of an orthopedic condition or arthritis in the hip can increase the possibility of a hip replacement.

9. **D** We do not know what causes psoriasis, and therefore, there is no cure. However, there are ways to treat it to make it feel better or to make it temporarily go away and be dormant. We do know that light aids in treatment.

10. **B** Because osteoporosis affects primarily the spine (even though the hip and other joints are affected), the vertebrae begin to collapse on top of each other. This is one reason why those with osteoporosis begin to lose height. This type of fracture is a compression fracture. Compound fractures break through the skin, comminuted are shattered breaks, and simple means simple break.

11. **D** Scleroderma has been found to be more common in women than in men.

12. **D** Since you are clean and already undressed, it is the better time. And children should also be checked since a cancerous mole found in adulthood could be treated in childhood if found to be pre-cancerous.

13. **C** Type I diabetes occurs when the pancreas is not functioning, which is why it is discovered generally at a young age (an organ not functioning will be noticeable). Type II is also known as adult onset. The problem here is the pancreas is producing the insulin; the body is just resisting it. Anemia refers to low iron levels.

14. **A** Insulin lowers blood sugar (which is why diabetics take it). If you wait all day to eat, anyone's blood sugar will drop, diabetic or not. The two combined will cause a diabetic's blood sugar to drop very low very quickly.

15. **B** The vena cavas drain blood into the heart. The atrium and ventricles of the heart are for blood, not lymph.

16. **C** Angioplasty is the surgical procedure to unclog an artery to the heart. Pericarditis is inflammation of the sac around the heart. Aneurysm is the bursting of a blood vessel. If an aneurysm occurs in the brain, it is called a stroke.

17. **C** Having a high HDL (high density lipoprotein) is a good thing, because this is the good cholesterol.

18. **A** Urine output increases with diabetes.

19. **A** Arterio means artery; sclerosis means hardening.

20. **A** If blood pressure is controlled, then it's not an issue. However, it is still best to consult with a physician since what he or she thinks is "controlled" may be different than the patient's definition.

21. **C** High blood sugar puts you at risk for diabetes and, therefore, heart disease, not low blood sugar.

22. **C** Fibromyalgia is an immune disorder but affects the muscles. Osteoporosis and osteoarthritis are bone disorders but are not immune disorders.

23. **C** When the myelin sheath begins to deteriorate, nerve impulses do not travel well down the nerve.

24. **B** Cystic fibrosis clients tend to have excess mucus and phlegm build up in their lungs. Tapotement and vibration will help loosen this some.

25. **B** Types of COPD include asthma, chronic bronchitis, and emphysema.

26. **C** This is the severe decrease in lateral rotation of the scapula.

27. **D** Angina pectoris is the medical term for chest pain. Myocardial infarction is the medical term for heart attack.

28. **A** Because of the pressure placed on the blood vessels with uncontrolled hypertension, the concern is an aneurysm in the brain also known as stroke or CVA.

29. **B** Since beta blockers (Tenormin, Lopressor, Atenolol) lower heart rate as well as BP, the concern is that the heart rate will lower while lying on a massage table and the client might feel dizzy when sitting or standing up.

30. **B** Aspirin can be for many things: pain, headache, blood thinner. Although D could be an answer because it does mask pain if that is what it is taken for, the bigger concern is the therapist's pressure for bruising.

31. **C** Congestive heart failure means blood is backing up in the heart and potentially the lungs. Massage may be a contraindication by the physician because of increasing the blood flow to a diseased heart that cannot pump this blood anywhere.

32. **B** "Negate" means negative or opposite of what is intended.

33. **B** Diagnosis is determining the disease; pathology is the study of disease; an anomaly is a disease that is irregular or different from the norm.

34. **A** Subjective means it is determined by the individual (objective means factual and observable). One person's pain tolerance is going to differ from another's.

35. **C** When exacerbated, it has reactivated or has gotten worse.

36. **B** Anomaly is a disease that is different from the norm; a placebo is something that possibly gives the desired affect because the client "thinks" it is real medicine but is not. Objective information will be taken by the doctor or nurse via blood pressure, X-rays, etc. (factual information).

37. **C** Benign means non-cancerous; chronic means the condition has been going on for a while and may have good/bad days but probably more bad. If it is chronic, it will take time to go away, but we do know from the client it is not contagious.

38. **A** Threshold is the minimal amount needed in order to produce the desired effect.

39. **D** Redness is the first stage. Vasodilation of the capillary walls allows blood plasma to merge into the interstitial spaces causing the increased swelling. The heat occurs because of the vasodilation.

40. **A** CAD stands for coronary artery disease (heart disease). Emphysema is a COPD (chronic obstructive pulmonary disease) and is not reversible.

41. **C** Diverticulosis is when food or a substance gets stuck in one of the crevices of the intestines and becomes infected. Liverenteritis is not a word.

42. **A** Gastroenteritis is an inflammation of the GI tract; diverticulitis is a disorder of the large intestines; and pleurisy is inflammation of the lungs.

43. **C** Pleurisy is inflammation of the tissue of the lungs; peritonitis is an inflammation of the lining of the abdomen; pericarditis is an inflammation of the sac around the heart; and diverticulitis is a disorder of the large intestines.

44. **A** Type I diabetes occurs when the pancreas is not functioning, which is why it is discovered generally at a young age (an organ not functioning will be noticeable). Type II is also known as adult onset, and the problem lies with the pancreas producing the insulin.

45. **D** Type I diabetes occurs when the pancreas is not functioning, which is why it is discovered generally at a young age (an organ not functioning will be noticeable). Type II is also known as adult onset. The problem here is that the pancreas is producing the insulin.

46. **C** Dialysis is a treatment to filter the blood because the kidneys are unable to do it themselves. Nephritis is a kidney disorder (the nephrons are located in the kidneys).

47. **B** This can occur especially with food allergies (peanuts, shellfish) and bee stings. It is life threatening.

48. **A** Media means middle (middle ear or inner ear), and oto means ear (otoscope allows the doctor to look into your ear).

49. **C** Driving habits may predispose someone to accidents but not disease.

50. **C** Embolism is a blood clot, and nephritis is inflammation of the kidneys (associated with the nephron).

51. **B** Cyanosis is bluish skin. Cystitis is a urinary tract infection. Conjunctiva is an eye infection.

52. **C** Angina means pain; pectoris means chest.

53. **B** Ortho means line or straight; static means stable; hypo means low; tension is associated with blood pressure. It is not contraindicated in massage unless it is due to another medical condition. However, people who normally have low blood pressure may have this. Remember, there are no cut-offs for low blood pressure, just high blood pressure (140/90).

54. **C** In torticollis, the head becomes extended forward and rotated or flexed.

55. **A** Virulent means the ability of an organism to cause a disease. Chronic means longer lasting.

56. **B** Cushing's disease is the secretion of too much adrenocorticotropic hormone. Hyperthyroidism is secretion of too much thyroid hormone; hypothyroidism is too little secretion. Diabetes is either no production of insulin or the body is resisting the insulin.

57. **C** Muscle pain is myalgia. Think of the term "fibromyalgia"; this is muscle fiber pain.

58. **D** Glaucoma is elevated pressure in the eye due to obstructed outflow of aqueous fluid. The lacrimal glands are the tear ducts.

59. **C** Impetigo is an inflammation of the skin caused by staph or strep bacteria. Psoriasis is red, flaky skin marked by periods of remission. Seborrhea is a topical disease of the skin where the oil glands are secreting too much sebum.

60. **D** Spasms of the bronchiole tubes is more related to asthma and bronchitis. Emphysema is rigidity of the respiratory muscles as well as the alveoli sacs inside the lungs which help with internal respiration dying off. Therefore, oxygen is blown out on exhalation instead of transported into the body.

61. **A** Osteoporosis is the loss of bone density. Rheumatoid arthritis is a systemic disease involving random inflammation that can also affect organs. Articulitis is a made-up word.

62. **C** Viruses do not respond to the treatment of antibiotics which is why we do not take them for colds.

63. **C** Pandemic is a disease that affects the entire world, such as AIDS.

64. **A** Virulent means extremely poisonous or harmful.

65. **C** While rheumatoid arthritis is an immune system disorder that may affect vital organs, it does not generally have a direct affect on the skin. Scleroderma is hardening of the skin and cells that line the digestive tract causing many nutritional problems as well as affecting other organs.

66. **A** This is where the mother can pass antibodies not only through the placenta but also through her breast milk to her child.

67. **D** This is why we get things such as redness or hives: from an allergic reaction.

68. **C** Cystitis is a urinary tract infection; nephritis is chronic inflammation of the kidneys; and hepatitis is a liver disorder.

69. **B** This is the basic definition for jock itch.

70. **C** Bell's palsy is a nerve disorder affecting cranial nerve VII that affects one side of the face. Alzheimer's affects the brain and its emotional/memory/thinking more so than the physical changes listed in this question. Senility is a term given to a variety of disorders and commonly associated with Alzheimer's.

71. **B** Impetigo is a bacterial infection of the skin; psoriasis is a noncontagious chronic skin disease with reddish patches; and seborrhea is a disease where the sebaceous glands increase the amount of oil substance released.

72. **C** Tendonitis is irritation to the tendon but not to a synovial sheath. A strain is a stretched or torn muscle or tendon; a sprain is a stretched or torn ligament.

73. **A** An avulsion occurs when the tendon tears away from the bone, sometimes taking a piece of the bone with it.

74. **C** Vaginitis is the irritation of the vagina; dysmenorrhea is menstrual pain; and endometriosis is abnormal cell growth of endometrial cells.

75. **B** High arches in the foot are called pes cavus; irritation of the plantar fascia is called plantar fasciitis.

76. **A** Myoma is a tumor in the muscle tissue; carcinoma is a cancerous area in the epithelial tissue; and lipoma is a fatty tumor.

77. **D** All of the choices listed can cause the spine to curve in a sideways manner.

78. **A** Decubitus ulcer is a medical term for bedsores that can be prevented if the patient is turned on a regular basis. They occur due to having to lie down (in bed) for a prolonged time.

79. **D** Phlebitis is irritation of veins; spider veins are the smaller bluish/purple veins; and venules are small veins.

80. **B** Spondylosis is osteoarthritis of the spine; semispinalis is a muscle of the back; and osteoarthritis is the wear-and-tear of the bones.

81. **B** ALS is also called Lou Gehrig's disease, after the famous baseball player, Lou Gehrig, who contracted the disease.

82. **D** These are the basic definition of contractures.

83. **A** Crohn's disease is an idiopathic condition usually of the small intestines, but sometimes of the large intestines. Abdominal massage is contraindicated although massage to areas outside of the abdomen is all right under the supervision of a physician.

84. **A** Pyelonephritis is an infection of the kidneys; peritonitis is inflammation of the abdominal lining; and peripheral vascular disease is a circulatory disease, but it does not necessarily make the client more sensitive to cold. It affects blood and lymph.

85. **A** Thoracic outlet syndrome can be caused not only by tight (hypertonic) scalenes, but structural abnormalities in the clavicle and the first and second ribs, too.

86. **C** Cyanosis is bluish skin. Tenosynovitis is inflammation of a tendon sheath; and spondylosis is osteoarthritis of the spine.

87. **A** Palpable is perception to touch, paresis is partial paralysis, and paraplegia is paralysis of both lower extremities.

88. **A** Diets low in iodine can also lead to thyroid disorders which is where a goiter is located.

89. **B** While all can be at risk, the ones who are most at risk are the postmenopausal due to the change in hormone levels.

90. **C** Rickets is characterized by defective bone growth and can also be due to lack of sun exposure.

91. **B** Disease is when the body is impaired physiologically and psychologically; a sprain is dealing with a ligament; anomaly is an abnormality.

92. **B** Ectopic pregnancy occurs when the fertilized egg does not settle in the uterus. This may occur in the fallopian tubes instead. Preeclampsia is a bacterial toxin in the blood and albumin in the urine that can complicate pregnancy. Spontaneous abortion can be caused by abruptio placentae.

93. **C** The area of psoriasis is contraindicated, but the other areas are not.

94. **B** Coming in contact with the disease makes it active; naturally acquired indicates there was no vaccine or any other artificial means of getting the immunity.

95. **A** A sprain is a torn or stretched ligament, and a strain is a torn or stretched tendon or muscle. A full and complete dislocation is a dislocation, but a partial is called a subluxation. Paridislocation is a made-up term.

96. **B** Kyphosis is the curvature of the thoracic spine. Because the client is elderly, this could be due to osteoporosis. Your best course of action is to get a doctor's clearance before massaging.

97. **C** Atrophy can be due to a disease, injury, or decrease in exercise. A body builder who quits training will atrophy his/her muscles, but it is not due to a disease or injury, it's from lack of training and the muscles getting smaller.

98. **A** Osteoporosis is generally due to lack of calcium; osteomalacia and rickets can be due to a lack of vitamin D.

99. **A** A fibroid is usually in the smooth muscle of the uterus. Although it can be very painful, it is generally benign.

100. **C** Although stress can cause hypertension, high blood pressure is the term. Cerebrovascular accident (CVA) is another term for stroke.

101. **C** Encephalitis is inflammation of the brain, and meningitis is inflammation of the meninges. Hydrocracialitis is a made-up term.

102. **B** This is a review of medical terminology.

103. **A** An embolus is a moving clot or air pocket; arteriosclerosis is hardening of the arteries; and parasthesia is the pins-and-needles feeling in an area of the body.

104. **A** Diverticulosis occurs when food or a substance gets stuck in one of the crevices of the intestines and becomes infected. Reflux is when stomach acid goes back up into the esophogus. Fundal ulcer is a made-up term.

105. **A** Graves' disease is due to too much thyroid hormone being released. Hypothyroidism is caused by too little hormone being released. Diabetes mellitus is characterized by glucose intolerance or deficiency. Cushing's disease is overproduction of adrenalcorticoid steroids.

106. **D** A sprain is a torn or stretched ligament, and a strain is a torn or stretched tendon or muscle.

107. **B** Physiology is the study of how the whole body and its parts function normally; psychology and psychiatry are studies of the normal and diseased mind.

108. **C** Physiotherapy is another term for physical therapy. Hydrotherapy is therapy using various means of water (steam, ice, heat). Psychiatry is therapy for mental illness.

109. **A** Relative means in relation to the disease or problem. Absolute means under no circumstances should a massage be given.

110. **B** Massage is contraindicated for phlebitis (inflammation of a vein) and thrombus (a blood clot).

111. **D** Ischemia is lack of oxygen; hypoxia is lack of oxygen; and anemia is lack of iron.

112. **A** "Hypo" means below, deep, under; subcutaneous means "under."

113. **C** Rheumatoid is an immune system disorder that shows itself through inflammation of joints or organs. Gout is uric acid crystal deposits usually in the big toe joint, and bursitis is irritation of the bursa sac.

114. **B** This is due to the blood pooling in the vein.

115. **B** Tendonitis is generally caused by overusing or repetitive movements to a tendon; migraines are vascular in nature; and CHF stands for chronic heart failure.

116. **C** This falls under the broad classification of arthritis.

117. **A** Rheumatoid is an immune system disorder that shows itself through inflammation of joints, organs, etc. Gout is uric acid crystal deposits usually in the big toe joint. Lupus is an immune disorder, and scleroderma literally means "hardening of the skin."

118. **B** Also, when the blood floods back into the right atrium, it can forcefully distend the atrium. If done enough, this would place undue stress on the heart and be especially risky for those with HBP and heart problems.

119. **A** We don't know why the vein is enlarged, and since it could be a clot that could be dislodged, we should not take the risk of massaging it.

120. **B** Eczema is crusty with watery discharge. Impetigo is caused by staph bacteria. Scleroderma is hardening of the skin.

121. **B** Bursitis and tendonitis are also inflammations, but do not necessarily mean there is a sprain or strain, or that the injury is chronic.

122. **C** Plantar warts are very painful.

123. **C** According to the American Heart Association, there are no cut-offs for low blood pressure as there are with HBP (which is 140/90), unless there is fainting, light-headedness, or dizziness for unknown reasons. This client does not, so she just has good BP. If it is below 120/70, doctors will state it is on the low side but not a health issue like HBP.

124. **C** Diabetes mellitus is a group of disorders that lead to elevated blood glucose. Diabetes insipidus does not have to do with blood sugar but with the levels of antidiuretic hormone (ADH).

125. **D** Dyspnea means unusual shortness of breath or difficulty breathing. Fatigue is a symptom of emphysema because the alveoli sacs that transport oxygen to the blood vessels are dying off, so not enough oxygen is getting to the organs and tissues. Loss of appetite occurs because eating is more difficult if you can't breathe well. Chronic cough is the fourth symptom and is not listed here.

126. **B** This is due to the cilia that are damaged from the smoke and carbon monoxide in cigarettes. The cilia then cannot get irritants and germs out of the airways. This causes inflammation of the tissues and eventually a breaking down of the elastic fibers in the respiratory system.

127. **A** COPD stands for chronic obstructive pulmonary disease and includes asthma, chronic bronchitis, and emphysema, but not cancer. The other terms are made up.

128. **B** Nephritis is inflammation of the kidneys. The other terms are made up.

129. **C** Hypoproteinemia is low blood protein; anemia is low iron in the blood; and reduced glomerular filtration is inefficient filtering of waste from the blood.

130. **D** Strokes usually affect one side causing hemiplegia, but the definition of the term is not "stroke."

131. **D** GERD stands for gastroesophogeal reflux disease and can cause shortness of breath because the nerve that innervates the esophogus innervates the trachea. When the esophogus closes off to try to control the stomach acid coming up, it closes off the trachea and affects breathing.

132. **D** Fewer than normal alveoli sacs is characteristic of emphysema

133. **A** It is a reflux (or reverse flow) of stomach acid into the esophagus, and it is a disease not a disorder.

134. **D** Although they can receive general massage, abdominal massage is contraindicated since

these are intestinal diseases that commonly have diarrhea as an effect.

135. **B** Obesity is a major risk factor, and too much estrogen has been shown to be a risk (this can be from pregnancy, hormone replacement, or birth control pills). Native Americans seem to have a higher risk because of a predisposition to secrete high levels of cholesterol in the bile, which explains the cholesterol choice as well.

136. **A** Hepatitis A is usually spread through food or water contaminated by feces. It usually resolves on its own over several weeks.

137. **A** Diabetes mellitus is a group of disorders that lead to elevated blood glucose. Gestational diabetes occurs during pregnancy but often goes away after delivery. Graves' disease is a thyroid disease, and diabetes insipidus is not related to blood sugar but to antidiuretic hormone levels.

138. **A** Also, decreased urination, dry skin, fatigue, light-headedness, and dark gold urine may be signs.

139. **C** Pruritus ani means itching, and fistulae are little tears that may occur around the anus.

140. **D** Because neurological function is affected, this would include the nerves to the intestines.

141. **C** Think about leukemia when the body starts fighting against its own immune system by forming too many leukocytes (white blood cells).

142. **C** This is the main reason for this contraindication. Remember, we do no harm. Massage could make the illness worse with infections.

143. **D** This is an inflammation of the veins, possibly systemically, and should be under the care of a physician.

144. **D** Massage is contraindicated for lupus.

145. **A** Because of the pressure placed on the blood vessels with uncontrolled hypertension, the concern is an aneurysm in the brain, also known as stroke or CVA.

146. **B** "Ipsa" means same; "contra" means opposite.

Therapeutic Massage and Bodywork Assessment

AREAS OF COMPETENCE

This chapter includes sections that correspond to the organization of the NCBTMB exam as follows:

NCETM (16%)   **NCETMB (18%)**

A. Assessment methods (visual, palpatory, auditory, olfactory, intuitive)
B. Assessing range of motion
C. Assessment areas (soft tissues and bony landmarks, endangerment sites, trigger points, adhesions, lymphatic edema, pulse rate)
D. Holding patterns (e.g., guarding, muscle/fascial memory)
E. Posture analysis
F. Structural and functional integration
G. Ergonomic factors
H. Effects of gravity
I. Proprioception of movement

Strategies to Success

Study Skills

Set goals!

The NCETM and NCETMB cover a lot of material, and it's not uncommon to feel stressed in trying to review it all. Try to make your workload easier by prioritizing and setting goals. Create a schedule to review material, and set aside time to practice answering exam questions. If there is a certain topic you know you have difficulty with, make sure you devote more time to review it and less time to something you already understand.

Assessment Methods

When working with a client, therapists and bodyworkers must evaluate each individual situation. Assessment is an ongoing information-gathering process that is used in making clinical decisions. While the pathology chapter helps to determine if a condition should be treated by massage, this chapter will discuss how to determine the best course of treatment. Table 4-1 presents various assessments methods. Table 4-2 presents the visual characteristics.

TABLE 4-1

At a Glance: Assessment Methods

HOPS

History	Includes the intake forms and medical clearance recommendations.
Observation	Includes postural analysis, visual cues, watching when your client does not know you are observing them so they do not make modifications.
Palpation	Assessment through touch and feel.
Special tests	Includes normal range of motion and measurements of postural analysis.

TABLE 4-2

At a Glance: Visual Assessment

Gait or walking pattern	Does the client take one normal step and one small step? Does the client swing only one arm? Is he/she compensating?
Posture	Is your client internally rotated at the shoulders? Does he/she have a forward head position? Does he/she have sway back?
Breathing patterns	Is your client using his/her diaphragm to breathe, or is he/she shoulder breathing?
Sympathetic or parasympathetic	Is the client in "fight or flight" mode or lethargic?

Normal Ranges of Motion

Combining postural analysis, information the client has given, and range of motion (ROM) assessment, the therapist can better assess injuries, muscular limitations, and weakness. Normal ranges of motion are noted below in Table 4-3. Range of motion limitations can be a sign of injury to the joint, muscle, tendons, or ligaments. If it is a joint or ligament structure, or if the tendon or muscle injury is severe or acute, referral is necessary. (For diagrams of the motions listed in table 4-3, refer to Chapter 2 pp. 48–51.)

TABLE 4-3

At a Glance: Normal Ranges of Motion	
Dorsiflexion of the foot	20–30 degrees
Plantar flexion of the foot	30–50 degrees
Inversion of the foot	50 degrees
Eversion of the foot	25 degrees
Flexion of the knee	160 degrees
Extension of the knee	180 degrees
Flexion of the hip	90 degrees if knee is extended; 120 degrees if knee is flexed
Extension of the hip	20 degrees
Medial/internal hip rotation	30 degrees
Lateral/external hip rotation	60 degrees
Abduction of the hip	45 degrees
Adduction of the hip	30 degrees
Flexion of the trunk	40–60 degrees
Extension of the trunk	35 degrees
Lateral flexion of the trunk	15–20 degrees
Rotation of the trunk	10–15 degrees in lumbar spine; 45 degrees in thoracic spine
Flexion of the neck	80 degrees
Extension of the neck	60–70 degrees
Lateral flexion of the neck	35–45 degrees
Rotation of the neck	80 degrees
Flexion of the shoulder	180 degrees
Extension of the shoulder	45–50 degrees
Abduction of the shoulder	180 degrees
Adduction of the shoulder	30–45 degrees
Medial/internal rotation of the shoulder	30–45 degrees
Lateral/external rotation of the shoulder	80 degrees
Horizontal abduction of the shoulder	30 degrees
Horizontal adduction of the shoulder	140 degrees

Endangerment Sites

Endangerment Sites:

Areas of the body are generally listed as endangerment sites if they have a major blood vessel (artery/vein), nerve, lymph nodes, organ, and/or sensitive bony landmark. These are areas that should be avoided due to the structures present in the area. However, for the low back, while this area can be massaged, vigorous tapotement should be avoided. Endangerment sites are listed below.

Anterior Triangle of the Neck

The borders of the anterior triangle of the neck are the trachea, base of the mandible, and the sternocleidomastoid.

- Common carotid arteries
- Hyoid bone
- Internal jugular vein
- Thyroid gland
- Trachea
- Vagus nerve
- Lymph nodes

Posterior Triangle of the Neck

The borders of the posterior triangle of the neck are the clavicle, the sternocleidomastoid, and the trapezius.

- Brachial plexus
- External jugular vein
- Facial nerve
- Subclavian artery
- Styloid process
- Lymph nodes

Axillary

- Axillary arteries and nerves
- Brachial arteries and plexus

- Median nerves
- Musculotaneous nerve
- Radial and ulnar nerve
- Personal space
- Axillary lymph nodes

Antecubital Area of Elbow

- Brachial artery
- Cubital vein
- Median nerve
- Radial/ulnar arteries

Femoral Triangle

The borders of the femoral triangle are the gracilis, sartorius, and inguinal ligament.

- Femoral artery and nerve
- Great saphenous vein
- Obturator nerve
- Inguinal lymph nodes

Low Back (Ribs Nine Through Twelve)

- Floating ribs
- Kidneys

Oleacronon Process Area

- Ulnar nerve
- Radial nerve

Popliteal Fossa

- Common peroneal nerves
- Popliteal arteries
- Tibial nerves

Postural Analysis

Postural analysis involves assessing the body's posture and related bone and muscle groups. Remember, when it comes to postural analysis, muscles can lie, but bones do not. Therefore, it is best to use bony landmarks for postural analysis whenever possible. Also remember to consider muscles above, below, and 360 degrees around the area of concern. Remember, it's all connected!

See the following list for items to include in a postural analysis.

1. Observation—either begin from the head down or the feet up. The client should be without shoes or socks. Things to look for include:
   A. Alignment of the Achilles tendon—Is the foot pronated, supinated, or neutral?
   B. Arches of the feet—You should be able to fit the distal phalange of the index finger under the arch. If you are unable to get that much under the arch, the client may have flat feet (pes planus); if more than that can go under the arch, the client may have high arches (pes cavas).
   C. Position of the feet—Are the hips medially or laterally rotated?
   D. Calf area—Is one larger than the other? Are they even?
   E. Popliteal fold—Is it level? If it is higher on the lateral side of the knee, it could indicated a tight (ITB) and/or anterior pelvic tilt.
   F. Hips—Are they level? If the hips are not level while the client is standing but are level when he/she is sitting, the problem is most likely below the hips. Is there an anterior or posterior tilt? See Figures 4-1 through 4-3. Check the level of the right anterior superior iliac spine (ASIS) compared to the right posterior superior iliac spine (PSIS) (also compare the left ASIS and the left PSIS). If the ASIS is five to ten degrees lower than the PSIS, the client has an anterior pelvic tilt. If the PSIS is lower than the ASIS at all, the client has a posterior pelvic tilt.

      Note: Women can have up to a five to ten degree anterior pelvic tilt and still be considered neutral.
   G. Spine—Is the client kyphotic in the thoracic region (exaggerated outward curve of the thoracic

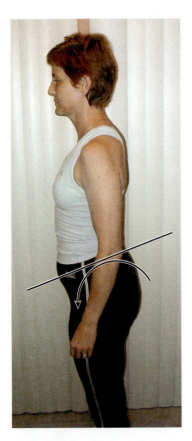

Figure 4-1 Anterior pelvic tilt.

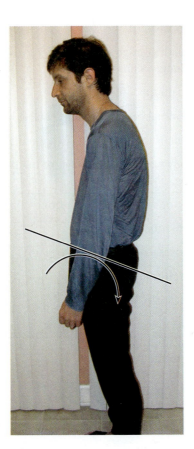

Figure 4-2 Posterior pelvic tilt.

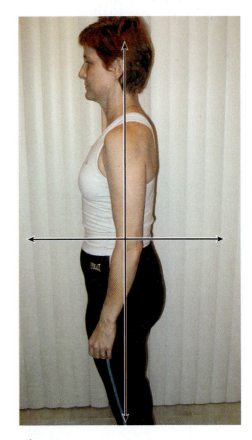

Figure 4-3 Neutral pelvic position.

spine), lordotic in the lumbar area (exaggerated inward curve or sway back), or scoliotic (sideways curve)? If there are curves, is it due to an anterior or posterior pelvic tilt or a high hip?

H. Shoulders/scapula—Are they even? Are they internally rotated?

I. Arms—Are the palms positioned to the side of the legs or to the front of the thigh (could indicate internal shoulder rotation)?

J. Head—Is it level, tilted to one side, or in a forward position?

See Table 4-4 for examples of muscles affected due to various postural abnormalities.

TABLE 4-4

At a Glance: Postural Abnormalites

Muscles that Are Shortened and Tight in a Posterior Pelvic Tilt	Gluteus maximus
	Hamstring group (semitendonosis, semimembranosis, biceps femoris)
	Gastrocnemius
	Soleus
	Rectus abdominus
	Weight tends to be shifted to the heels of the feet, so the heels of the feet may be tender.
Muscles that Are Shortened and Tight in an Anterior Pelvic Tilt	Sartorius
	Iliopsoas
	Quadriceps group (rectus femoris, vastus medialis, vastus intermedialis, vastus lateralis)
	Quadratus lumborum
	Iliotibial band and tensor fascia latae
	Tibialis anterior (increases likelihood of shin splints)
	Body weight tends to be on the balls of the feet and therefore may be tender.
Muscles that Are Shortened and Tight in Internal Shoulder Rotation	Pectoralis major and minor
	Latissimus dorsi
	Subscapularis
	Serratus anterior
	Sternocleidomastoid
	Scalenes

Understanding Kinesiology

In Chapter 2, kinesiology was defined as the study of body movement. Remember, in assessing muscles that are tight and shortened rather than taut and stretched, the therapist needs to understand postural analysis. Tight muscles are overly shortened, while taut muscles are overly stretched. The body itself works as a pulley system. If muscles on the anterior side are shortened and tight, the muscles opposite must be lengthened and taut. These lengthened and taut muscles still need work for possible trigger points, but the focus of the massage should be to loosen the shortened and tight muscles to help re-educate them for proper position and function. For example, many clients come to therapists with upper back and neck pain and want nothing but upper back and neck work. In performing a postural analysis, the therapist may find that the client is internally rotated. That would mean pecs, lats, and other anterior muscles must be worked. Trigger points may exist in the lengthened muscles (trapezius, rhomboids, and serratus posterior superior) and still need to be released, but the focus of the work would be on the muscles of internal shoulder rotation to help release somatic holding patterns.

Somatic holding patterns: Skeletal muscles are contracted based on the golgi tendon/muscle spindle reflex discussed in Chapters 1 and 2. Unfortunately, some of us are constantly in "fight-or-flight" mode, causing these holding patterns to create muscular issues and pain. Somatic pain comes from the stimulation of receptors in the skin, skeletal muscles, joints, tendons, and fascia. Ergonomic factors play a large role in these somatic holding patterns.

Other Factors that Affect the Body

Ergonomics: Ergonomics is the study of the anatomy, physiology, and psychology of how the body adjusts to the environment and equipment used in activity. For example, the body will adapt to computer use through correct or incorrect posturing. Massage therapists and bodyworkers generally see the client when incorrect ergonomics are being used and problems occur. For example, we know the proper way to lift an object from the floor, but habit has taught our muscles to do it wrong. Stabilizers (the back muscles) become primary movers, and we end up getting hurt.

But if we look at toddlers, they naturally pick things up from the floor using proper techniques. We educate our bodies and muscles to perform tasks incorrectly, maybe because we are in a hurry and it is easier at the time. However, over a period of time, our muscles are abused until one day the muscles cannot take it anymore. Thus, we injure our back, our neck, our knees, and so on. So we go to the therapist/bodyworker, and he/she checks our posture, noting that we have curves, tilts, and other abnormalities due to muscle tightness or guarding patterns. The therapist must now use that postural analysis and knowledge of muscle origins, insertions, and actions to determine which muscles are tight versus lengthened. The therapist works these muscles, stretches them, and uses other techniques such as heat or energy work. The therapist also assigns the client stretches to perform at home in order to continue the re-education of these muscles. As the muscles become re-educated, the client has now developed a kinesthetic or proprioceptive sense of when his/her body is not in correct position and can make appropriate adjustments.

Proprioception: Proprioception is knowing where the body is in relation to space (see Chapter 1). In other words, if you close your eyes and hold your arm out at shoulder length, the muscle spindles, golgi tendons, and other receptors send messages to and from the brain to let you know that your arm is indeed at shoulder level without having to look at it. Elderly people sometimes lose this ability, which is why they sometimes look at their feet when they walk. Eyes, ears, and other special senses also play a role in proprioceptive skills.

Gravity: Gravity is the force that keeps us on the ground. It can work with us or against us. Because of the curves of our spine and the structure of our bodies, when muscles become weak, gravity puts undue stress on various muscles and joints. This is why we need to be not only flexible but also strong. As massage therapists and bodyworkers, there are several things you can do to lengthen your careers and reduce the risk of injuries:

- check the massage table height
- wear comfortable attire that you can easily move in
- warm up and stretch before and after giving massages
- use a variety of strokes
- position your pressure so that you are behind your work
- maintain proper body mechanics
- breathe
- move smoothly
- get in tune with your body

Strategies to Success

Test-Taking Skills

Don't leave any questions blank!

Make an educated guess for every question even if you don't know the right answer. There is no penalty for guessing, and you might get a few extra points just by filling in every bubble.

*Some questions are not directly addressed in this chapter, but are meant to act as a general review of subjects studied in various school curriculums.

Questions

Therapeutic Massage Assessments
NCETM (16%) NCETMB (18%)

1. When massaging a child
   A. use towels as a top drape only.
   B. obtain written consent from both parents and child.
   C. have a parent supervise the massage session.
   D. ask the parent or guardian to wait outside the massage room.

2. A client with lordosis may experience a reduction in low back discomfort if a pillow is placed
   A. under the abdomen in the prone position.
   B. under the chest in the prone position.
   C. under the pelvis in the prone position.
   D. None of the above are correct.

3. In choosing the right kind of table, which of the following is not important?
   A. color
   B. comfort
   C. ergonomics
   D. ease of adjustment

4. Avoid massaging a new scar, especially after surgery, for
   A. seventy-two hours.
   B. one to two weeks.
   C. six to eight weeks.
   D. six months.

5. The goal of postural analysis is
   A. to evaluate current problems.
   B. to prevent future problems.
   C. to provide information to correct problems.
   D. All of the above are correct.

6. The type of muscle soreness caused by tiny microscopic tears in the muscle is called
   A. DOMS.
   B. day of muscle soreness.
   C. cyriax.
   D. Both A and B are correct.

7. An injury where a tendon is partially torn is called
   A. a sprain.
   B. myalgia.
   C. a strain.
   D. a rupture.

8. You have an athlete who is a basketball player coming to you because of calf pain. Because of the type of activity, you believe the problem is due to
   A. excessive force due to eccentric contractions on the gastrocnemius.
   B. excessive force due to concentric contractions on the gastrocnemius.
   C. excessive force due to isokinetic force on the gastrocemius.
   D. None of the above are correct.

9. Assessment of an athlete should occur during
   A. intercompetition massage and post-event massage.
   B. pre-event massage and post-event massage.
   C. pre-event massage and intercompetition massage.
   D. post-event massage only.

10. Early warning signs of overtraining include all of the following EXCEPT
    A. insomnia.
    B. washed-out feeling.
    C. lower than normal blood pressure.
    D. insatiable thirst.

11. When using proper body mechanics during a massage, your body weight should be in what area to reduce injuries to the knees the
    A. balls of the feet.
    B. abdomen.
    C. knees.
    D. heels of the feet.

12. When performing massage, your strength and pressure should come from
    A. your legs.
    B. your arms.
    C. your shoulders.
    D. None of the above are correct.

13. If a client has osteoporosis, what modifications (if any) should be made for his or her massage?
    A. deeper tissue work is warranted
    B. lighter tissue work is necessary
    C. range of motion stretches are most beneficial
    D. trigger point therapy would be beneficial

14. If a client is prone to heartburn, your recommendation would be
    A. check with physician before receiving a massage.
    B. do not eat a large meal before massage.
    C. abdominal massage is contraindicated.
    D. All of the above are correct.

15. Your client states that he or she is constipated. Your recommendation is
    A. abdominal massage is contraindicated.
    B. abdominal massage is indicated.
    C. full body massage is contraindicated.
    D. see a physician before any massage.

16. Your client has rheumatoid arthritis. She calls you to set up an appointment for today because she is having a flare-up in her knee. Your response is
    A. I can see you, but I will need to avoid your knee that's inflamed.
    B. I can see you and we will focus on your knee to get the swelling down.
    C. I cannot see you because your whole body is affected by your flare-up.
    D. I cannot see you since we cannot massage your knee; we might as well wait to do a full body massage.

17. Name the sharp protuberance on the inferior aspect of the temporal bone.
    A. coranoid
    B. styloid
    C. coracoid
    D. pterygoid

18. Massage has been shown to be beneficial to those who are paralyzed or injured to the point that they cannot use a limb. This is because massage can
    A. stimulate the parasympathetic nervous system.
    B. improve circulation and muscle tone through effleurage and petrissage.
    C. increase flexibility in these clients.
    D. increase nerve sensations.

19. The main source of a massage therapist's pressure should come from the
    A. hands.
    B. arms.
    C. back.
    D. lower body.

20. An eating disorder is characterized as
    A. a psychological disorder observed as an obsession with food/weight.
    B. easily treatable with a registered/licensed dietician.
    C. not a life-threatening disorder.
    D. generally only focuses on food but not exercise addiction.

21. Massage is indicated for which condition?
    A. acute ankle sprain
    B. pleurisy
    C. spider veins
    D. varicose veins

22. What should you do if a client states on his or her intake form that they have low blood pressure?
    A. get a physician's release before massaging him or her
    B. massage lightly
    C. emphasize the strokes in the caudal direction
    D. there are no contraindications

23. If a client tells you he or she cannot sleep on his or her back without a pillow under his or her knees, you the therapist may need to focus on what area of the body during his or her massage?
    A. knees
    B. iliopsoas
    C. hamstrings
    D. erector spinae

24. Endangerment sites include all of the following except
    A. medial brachium.
    B. upper lumbar region.
    C. anterior to the ear.
    D. ulnar notch.

25. Which of the following demonstrates good body mechanics?
    A. balance on both feet while leaning from the waist
    B. knees bent while keeping the back straight and lunging forward
    C. arms close to the body while shoulders are extended
    D. wrist extended fully

26. When massaging a client with Bell's palsy, what area of the body should be massaged with caution?
    A. inferior to the ear
    B. posterior triangle of the neck
    C. anterior to the ear
    D. superior to the ear

27. Tendonitis is defined best as a/an
    A. acute injury.
    B. overuse injury.
    C. sprain.
    D. nerve impingement.

28. If a condition is contraindicated for massage, it means
    A. to proceed with caution.
    B. requires medical attention, but proceed with the massage.
    C. do not perform the massage.
    D. the condition requires medication.

29. The reason that massage is contraindicated in cases of intoxication is
    A. massage can spread toxins and overwork the liver.
    B. the client may pass out on your table.
    C. the client's sensitivity to pain is lessened.
    D. the client may pursue inappropriate behavior.

30. When massaging an injured limb, it is best to
    A. massage over the injury.
    B. massage distal to the injury.
    C. massage proximal to the injury.
    D. perform friction on the injury.

31. The ability of the muscles, joints, and nerves to function well with one another for a common good is called
    A. balance and flexibility.
    B. health and fitness.
    C. grounding and centering.
    D. chi.

32. Poor working posture and hand technique can increase the risk of
    A. fibromyalgia.
    B. Epstein-Barre Syndrome.
    C. carpal tunnel syndrome.
    D. lordosis.

33. Mild dryness of the skin on a client
    A. should be avoided.
    B. is an absolute contraindication.
    C. benefits from massage due to increased sebum production.
    D. None of the above are correct.

34. Which one of the following is not an endangerment site?
    A. femoral triangle
    B. brachial plexus
    C. coracoid process
    D. styloid process of the temporal bone

35. The SOAP note format is also used in report writing. A report that covers the period from prescription through the first session is known as
    A. initial evaluation.
    B. status report.
    C. progress report.
    D. subjective report.

36. When addressing pressure with the client during the massage, it is helpful to
    A. ask the client to simply raise a hand if pain is felt.
    B. use the one to five point scale where one is no pain and five is excruciating pain.
    C. ask the client to stand as much discomfort as possible, especially when doing deep tissue work.
    D. Both A and B are correct.

37. The therapist may refuse to massage in part or in total a client based on
    A. the physical appearance or behavior of the client.
    B. information gleaned through the health history.
    C. inappropriate language.
    D. All of the above are correct.

38. Which of the following sensations are not associated with the trigger point referred sensation phenomenon?
    A. aching or pain
    B. tingling or numbness
    C. intense itching
    D. burning

39. To aid in your client's comprehension of directions during the massage, it is often best to
    A. use tactile cues and gestures.
    B. talk louder.
    C. keep going.
    D. use questions written on note cards.

40. The most frequent complaint that athletes bring to a massage therapist is
    A. injuries.
    B. muscle soreness.
    C. strength issues.
    D. adhesions.

41. Which statement is false?
    A. spasms and trigger points can create an environment in which lesions are more likely to occur
    B. the closer to a period of physical exertion, the less intrusive the sports massage should be
    C. compression is designed to create ischemia in sports massage
    D. the repair response in the soft tissues of the body is an example of homeostasis

42. Which of the following is not a warning sign of overtraining?
    A. insomnia
    B. low resting pulse
    C. elevated BP
    D. fatigue

43. Sports massage should be tailored to meet the needs of the
    A. athletic trainer.
    B. coach.
    C. team.
    D. athlete.

44. The tracking response in sports massage is
    A. finding bands of tension that inhibit performance.
    B. what happens when an athlete overtrains.
    C. what happens when an athlete undertrains.
    D. observing a client's reaction to a technique.

45. Which of the following is an important factor to consider when examining an athlete's training program?
    A. intensity of the workout
    B. frequency and duration
    C. athlete's goals
    D. All of the above are correct.

46. One of the most common chronological scenarios that athletes regularly report is
    A. tendon pain that subsides when they begin activity.
    B. better sleep without exercise.
    C. less DOMS with more fruit.
    D. decreased flexibility when not properly hydrated.

47. Which of the following is not a factor to consider when determining scheduling and technique selection for sports massage?
    A. amount of massage experience the athlete has had
    B. familiarity between the athlete and the therapist
    C. what the athlete ate for his/her last meal
    D. individual responsiveness to various approaches and techniques

48. Table height considerations include
    A. the height of the therapist.
    B. the thickness of the client when lying on the table.
    C. the type of technique used, such as deep pressure.
    D. All of the above are correct.

49. The ability to carry out daily tasks efficient with enough energy left over to enjoy leisure pursuits is called
    A. stamina.
    B. exercise.
    C. fitness.
    D. health.

50. A major focus for massage performance enhancement and injury prevention is
    A. appropriate sleep.
    B. always use heel of hand friction.
    C. take dietary supplements.
    D. None of the above are correct.

51. Which of the following is not a cause of delayed muscle soreness?
    A. pain-spasm-pain
    B. connective tissue damage
    C. adhesions
    D. damaged nerves

52. The intent of maintenance massage in sports massage is to
    A. enhance performance.
    B. locate cause of injury.
    C. implement self-care on the athlete.
    D. All of the above are correct.

53. The speed at which tissue repair occurs depends on
    A. the client's compliance regarding self-care.
    B. the extent of the injury.
    C. the frequency and nature of treatment.
    D. All of the above are correct.

54. As pressure is being applied, it is often helpful to watch the client's face for distortions to know if the pressure is too much. Another way to tell is the
    A. client's breathing pattern changes.
    B. client is asleep.
    C. client sighs.
    D. tissue relaxes.

55. A way to tell if a client might have a tight piriformis is to look at him or her to see if
    A. his or her hip/foot is externally rotated when he or she stands.
    B. his or her hip/foot is internally rotated when he or she stands.
    C. if his or her knee lifts up when the opposite leg is lifted to ninety degrees.
    D. if he or she has a posterior pelvic tilt.

56. What primary function(s) do universal precautions serve?
    A. protect the client and therapist
    B. protect the client from the therapist
    C. protect the state and the county
    D. protect the therapist from the client

57. Areas of the body where a bodyworker may compress a blood vessel or nerves is called a/an
    A. trigger point.
    B. tender point.
    C. endangerment site.
    D. tsubo.

58. In order to relax the pectoralis major on your client, the best position would be
    A. client supine with pillow under the head.
    B. client supine with a pillow under the arm(s).
    C. client prone with pillow under the abdomen.
    D. None of the above are correct.

59. A red, swollen, hot ankle would be classified as
    A. acute.
    B. subacute.
    C. chronic.
    D. third degree strain.

60. It is best to rotate the head ipsilaterally when working the sternocleidomastoid muscle (SCM) in order to
    A. work deeper on the muscle.
    B. make the client comfortable.
    C. avoid the carotid.
    D. avoid the popliteal plexus.

61. Massage below the navel is contraindicated for
    A. constipation.
    B. ethicality.
    C. bladder infection.
    D. All of the above are correct.

62. The most common cause of tendonitis is
    A. degeneration.
    B. overuse.
    C. injury.
    D. ligament damage.

63. The most potent technique in the therapeutic use of cold is to combine it with heat. This is called
    A. cryokinetics.
    B. cold mitten friction.
    C. hot and cold friction.
    D. contrast bath.

64. Your client has come to you with a shoulder bursitis. You should
    A. perform light massage on the shoulder.
    B. perform neuromuscular therapy (NMT) on the rotator cuff.
    C. recommend heat.
    D. refer to the doctor.

65. Your client comes to you asking you to work on a surgical scar that has pain near it. Your best action is to
    A. use friction on the scar to break up adhesions.
    B. use deep effleurage to move stagnant lymph.
    C. use petrissage to lift muscle away from the adhesions.
    D. refer to the doctor.

66. A common indication for abdominal massage is
    A. diverticulitis.
    B. hiatal hernia.
    C. constipation.
    D. All of the above are correct.

67. Which endanger site is located on the anterior elbow?
    A. cubital vein
    B. jugular vein
    C. popliteal artery
    D. radial process

68. Which of the following assesses the joint or ligament involvement in pain and the limitation of movement?
    A. active range of motion
    B. passive range of motion
    C. manual resistance
    D. proprioneuromuscular facilitation (PNF)

69. Just below ribs nine to twelve on the posterior side of the body is an endangerment site because
    A. the renal artery is located there.
    B. the renal nerve is located there.

C. the kidneys are located there.
    D. it is not an endangerment site.

70. The best method to determine weakness in muscles is to use
    A. passive ROM.
    B. active ROM.
    C. manual resistance.
    D. weight machines.

71. Your client comes to you with a headache, nausea, and drowsiness. You should
    A. do the massage focusing on occipitalis.
    B. do the massage focusing on splenius capitus.
    C. do the massage focusing on Swedish.
    D. Do not do the massage.

72. For post-fracture and amputation stumps, massage is
    A. by physician referral only.
    B. indicated.
    C. absolute contraindication.
    D. relative contraindication.

73. The most important aspect of the plan section in the SOAP notes is
    A. establishing a timeline for therapy.
    B. follow-up and evaluation of therapy.
    C. management of goals to produce the desired outcomes.
    D. reminders and session notes.

74. What bony landmark is near an endangerment site?
    A. medial epicondyle
    B. C7
    C. tibial tuberosity
    D. gluteal tuberosity

75. Another name for a scrape on the skin is a/an
    A. contusion.
    B. abrasion.
    C. contracture.
    D. bruise.

76. Your client comes to you with a bruise on the skin and a large lump underneath. He or she said he or she fell several weeks ago. What should you do?
    A. massage the area to decrease the lump
    B. avoid the area
    C. not perform the massage at all
    D. None of the above are correct.

77. Your client comes to you stating that he or she is so tight, he or she cannot touch his or her toes. He or she says the hamstrings are tight. You find that it is the quads. How could you tell?
    A. he or she has a posterior pelvic tilt
    B. one iliac crest is higher than the other
    C. he or she has a high shoulder
    D. he or she has an anterior pelvic tilt

78. Your client is slumped forward and his or her palms are facing the sides of his or her legs. This might indicate
    A. tight pectoralis major.
    B. tight latissimus dorsi.
    C. kyphosis of the spine.
    D. Both A and B are correct.

79. Your client feels pain behind the patella. This might mean he or she has
    A. a cartilage tear.
    B. chondromalacia.
    C. patellar tendonitis.
    D. a ligament sprain.

80. A home therapy program for a client must be
    A. too challenging.
    B. too easy so they will do it.
    C. time-consuming.
    D. None of the above are correct.

81. A prescription from a doctor for a client to receive massage therapy that will be submitted to insurance for reimbursement should include
    A. frequency of sessions per week.
    B. total number of sessions.
    C. length of session.
    D. All of the above are correct.

82. For the client with asthma, muscles to focus on include all of the following except
    A. intercostals.
    B. levator scapula.
    C. trapezius.
    D. latissimus dorsi.

83. An elderly man tells you he has had a left swollen ankle for two weeks. You should
    A. use the RICE principle.
    B. refer him to a doctor.
    C. use lymphatic drainage.
    D. use light effleurage.

84. In treating kyphosis, the goal is to relax and stretch which muscle?
    A. rhomboids
    B. pectoralis major
    C. erector spinae
    D. All of the above are correct.

85. Clients reporting on their problems, beliefs, attitudes, and biases goes in which section of the SOAP notes?
    A. subjective
    B. objective
    C. action
    D. plan

86. If a client comes to you with a second degree cervical sprain, you should
    A. focus on the anterior neck muscles.
    B. not work on the neck at all because it is contraindicated.
    C. wait until the acute injury is in the chronic phase to work on it.
    D. massage as usual.

87. Updating the client's "S" note in SOAPs before the start of the following session is necessary for
    A. determining the effect of the previous session.
    B. determining if the massage plan needs adjustment.
    C. determining if the client was satisfied.
    D. Both A and B are correct.

88. The primary thing to keep in mind when planning therapy goals is to
    A. remain flexible.
    B. use published studies.
    C. remain constant.
    D. All of the above are correct.

89. Your client fell while getting out of the bathtub. She fell straight back and landed on her back. Now her lower back is hurting with pain over the PSIS. What might be the problem?
    A. she bruised her tailbone
    B. she has SI joint dysfunction
    C. she damaged the sacrotuberous ligament
    D. she tightened the psoas and tore fibers

90. Your client complains that her knee feels like it is locking up on her or that it gives way. This is a sign of
    A. torn cartilage.
    B. torn ACL.
    C. torn patellar tendon.
    D. chondromalacia.

91. Pes cavas is another term for
    A. loss of the longitudinal arch in the foot.
    B. loss of the transverse arch in the foot.
    C. high arch in the foot.
    D. low arch in the foot.

92. A method of communication should be established with the client before starting a chair massage because
    A. it is so different from table massage.
    B. eye contact is not possible.
    C. communication is not important in chair because it is almost impossible to hurt someone.
    D. Both A and B are correct.

93. When evaluating a client with an injury, it is best to test the uninjured side due to all of the following except
    A. increased trust in the therapist.
    B. decreased fear of the unknown for the client.
    C. increased muscle guarding.
    D. providing a baseline for comparison.

94. Information assessed and documented by visual observation includes all of the following except
    A. gait.
    B. muscle spasm.
    C. skin integrity.
    D. mental status.

95. The problem of Morton's toe is
    A. the first toe is shorter than the second.
    B. the second toe is longer than the first.

C. the nerve between the third and fourth metatarsal is inflamed.
    D. None of the above are correct.

96. Bunionettes are generally located on the
    A. side of the big toe.
    B. side of the little toe.
    C. heel.
    D. ball of the foot.

97. Your client says her doctor told her she has a dropped transverse arch in her foot. This means she will have
    A. flat feet.
    B. high arches.
    C. splayed toes.
    D. None of the above are correct.

98. Thoracic outlet syndrome mimics
    A. whiplash.
    B. torticollis.
    C. carpal tunnel syndrome.
    D. All of the above are correct.

99. Another term for pes planus is
    A. flat feet.
    B. high arches.
    C. lost transverse arch.
    D. None of the above are correct.

100. Information assessed and documented primarily by palpatory observation includes all of the following except
    A. location of the muscles.
    B. identification of the soft tissue problem.
    C. postural symmetry.
    D. response to pressure.

Answers and Explanations

Therapeutic Massage Assessments
NCETM (16%) NCETMB (18%)

1. **C** The best and safest thing to do for both child and therapist is to have a parent in the room during the massage session.

2. **A** This will help to lengthen the low back and put the client in a more neutral pelvic position which would be more comfortable. Remember, lordosis is sway back.

3. **A** As much as we decide on the color of our tables, they are covered up by the sheets!

4. **C** This allows time for the scar to heal but not so long that adhesions would appear deep in the tissue.

5. **D** Postural analysis is utilizing bony landmarks to determine postural abnormalities that are or could cause problems down the road for your client, such as high hips and anterior pelvic tilts. Knowing what specific muscles are the tight ones helps the therapist to focus on the best therapies.

6. **A** DOMS stands for **D**elayed **O**nset **M**uscle **S**oreness and is generally characterized by tiny microscopic tears.

7. **C** Strains occur in muscles and tendons (the "T" in strain, and the "T" in tendon may help you remember). Sprains occur in ligaments (a sprained ankle). Myalgia means muscle pain. A rupture is a complete, not partial, tear of a muscle or tendon.

8. **A** The landing phase of the jump is an eccentric (lengthening yet contracting) effect on the gastrocnemius. Eccentric contractions place more force on the muscle because the external force (gravity in this case) is greater than the muscular force. Therefore, eccentric contractions can cause more injuries.

9. **D** The pre-event and intercompetition should be used to focus on preparing the athlete for competition and psyching them up. Telling them they have a problem viewed in your assessment at either one of these times may cause the athlete to lose focus and not perform well.

10. **C** Blood pressure elevates because the body is not able to recover, creating a "stress" situation.

11. **D** If weight is placed on the balls of the feet, the knees go in front of the toes during lunging. This places stress directly on the knee joint, causing problems. With the weight on the heels of the feet, weight is placed on the leg muscles, which is better and safer.

12. **A** Raising the table may create shoulder and neck problems. Standing up straighter places more stress on the hands, wrist, elbows, and shoulders for pressure; straightening the knees places more stress on the back. Therefore, lowering the table and getting into a better lunge allows for the back to be in a better mechanical position with pressure coming from the legs.

13. **B** Since osteoporosis is brittle bones, lighter pressure should be used. Too much pressure over bones or on the muscles that attach to the affected bones can create stress fractures in an already weakened bone.

14. **B** Eating a large meal then lying flat on the back can cause the stomach acid to reflux (go up into the esophagus), activating the heartburn.

15. **B** Abdominal massage is wonderful for the potential relief of constipation.

16. **C** Rheumatoid arthritis is an immune system disorder that shows itself through inflammation of joints and organs. Even though you are physically seeing the flare-up in one location, the flare-up is affecting everything inside the body. Also, it is acute, and bodyworkers do not work on acute.

17. **B** This is also an endangerment site.

18. **B** Studies have shown that working the unaffected limb can send similar neurological impulses to the injured side. Also, if given doctor's approval, working the affected side will still help manually move blood and lymph towards the heart to improve circulation.

19. **D** Proper mechanics help ensure a longer career.

20. **A** Eating disorders are psychological disorders that are visually seen as an eating disorder. The client has generally gone through or is going through much more than an obsession with weight or appearance; many times it is a control issue due to lost or lack of control in other areas of his or her life. A dietitian is very important in his or her treatment; however, a psychologist/psychiatrist is also necessary. Also, overexercising is a way of "purging" food.

21. **C** The ankle sprain is acute, and body workers do not work on acute injuries (new ones). Pleurisy is an infection of the fluid of the lung tissue (pleural sacs), so work is contraindicated. Varicose veins are where the valves in the veins do not function properly, and blood pools in the lower extremities. Massage can further damage these vessels.

22. **D** The American Heart Association as well as other organizations do not have cut-offs for low blood pressure like they do for high blood pressure. Therefore, generally, there are no contraindications to activities of daily living which would include massage and exercise.

23. **B** Your client is letting you know that for him or her to lie with his or her knees straight, his or her back hurts. This may indicate an anterior pelvic tilt (the back is arched and unsupported with the knees straight in the supine position). This would mean focusing on iliopsoas, rectus femoris, and quadratus lumborum. Iliopsoas is the only answer choice listed.

24. **C** Inferior to the ear would have made "C" an endangerment site due to the styloid process, but anterior to the ear is not an endangerment site.

25. **B** "B" is better mechanically since this reduces stress to the back, wrist, and shoulders.

26. **A** This is due to the facial nerve coming out between the mastoid process and the styloid process, both inferior to the ear.

27. **B** Tendonitis is generally caused by overusing or repetitive movements to a tendon.

28. **C** Contraindicated means "opposite" (contra) of indicated.

29. **A** While the other three choices may occur, the main reason is that the liver will be overworked; this can cause medical problems down the road.

30. **C** Proximal to the injury puts you closer to the midline and closer to the heart and lymph system. This will allow any metabolic waste to be put into circulation, so the body can rid itself of it and progress the healing process.

31. **A** This includes strength, flexibility, endurance, and proprioception.

32. **C** Fibromyaliga and Epstein-Barre are immune-system related. Carpal tunnel is a repetitive stress injury.

33. **C** Massage increases sebum production which would help MILD skin dryness.

34. **C** The coracoid process is part of the scapula and has the attachments of biceps brachii, pec minor, and coracobrachialis.

35. **A** Initial means beginning.

36. **D** "No pain, no gain" is not true. If too much pain is felt, the muscles will respond by tightening up more, which is not what you want.

37. **D** These are basic screening techniques.

38. **C** These are basic trigger point sensations.

39. **A** Remember the client may be relaxed, asleep, hard of hearing, and many other things, so tactile cues and gestures would be best.

40. **B** This is due to repetitive training and level of intensity.

41. **C** You do not want to create ischemia because that creates lack of blood flow. Our job is to increase blood flow.

42. **B** Because the body is under "stress" it cannot recover from day-to-day training; the resting pulse begins to go up.

43. **D** With the athletic trainer's approval, the massage is to benefit the client, which in this case is the athlete.

44. **B** Sometimes a "band" can be several areas that are related to one movement that can limit flexibility and performance.

45. **D** Since an athlete may be overtraining, leading to more injuries or not recuperating well, it's important to look at all of these. The same can be said for undertraining.

46. **D** Hydration can affect many things including the muscle function, whether it's strength, power, endurance, or flexibility.

47. **A** Massage experience is not a factor in scheduling.

48. **D** These are all important considerations for table height.

49. **C** Fitness is defined as this, but health is dealing with disease. One can be fit and still be unhealthy because of a disease. One can be healthy and still be unfit.

50. **B** Heel of hand friction is best to use on overuse injuries.

51. **D** Think of the definition of DOMS.

52. **A** That is why we call it "performance massage."

53. **D** All are factors in rehabilitation.

54. **A** Changes in breathing can indicate too much pressure, such as when the breath is held.

55. **A** The action of the piriformis is external hip rotation, so if it is tight, the foot and hip will be turned outward.

56. **A** "A" is the better answer. "C" is not relative since the concern is not for governments; the concern is the people coming in contact with each other.

57. **C** These are areas that should be avoided because of the nerve, blood vessel, or lymph nodes.

58. **B** Since the pectoralis major attaches to the humerus, supporting under the arm will help relax the muscle.

59. **A** If it is red and swollen, it is a new injury or a new flare-up and would be classified as acute.

60. **C** This allows the therapist to avoid the carotid easily and safely.

61. **C** To work the rectus abdominus, the therapist (with client knowledge and permission) would need to work below the navel almost down to the pubis symphysis. Therefore, ethical issues are not the concern here. Abdominal massage is wonderful for constipation, but the bladder infection is still an infection, and these should not be massaged.

62. **B** Tendonitis is generally caused by overusing or repetitive movements to a tendon.

63. **D** This is a review of hydrotherapy.

64. **D** Because massage cannot help in an acute bursitis, the best thing is for the client to see a physician to rule out anything else, rest it, and, when the inflammation comes down, begin light work.

65. **D** Pain on or near a surgical scar needs medical attention.

66. **C** Diverticulitis is an inflammation and infection of the pockets of the large intestines. Hiatal hernia is the protrusion of an organ through connective tissue.

67. **A** The jugular vein is in the neck near the carotid; the popliteal artery is behind the knee; and the radial process is not an endangerment location.

68. **B** The more relaxed the client is, the more accurate your assessment will be. The more active they are, the more guarding there is, and the more likely you will get a false negative test.

69. **C** This is a review of endangerment sites.

70. **C** Having the client resist against you and your resistance allows you to compare left and right sides; using weight machines is out of our scope of work.

71. **D** Drowsiness is the key factor; it could be something more than a headache and needs further investigation by a physician.

72. **B** At this point, a client is no longer under the care of a physician for these situations.

73. **C** The "plan" includes goals. While the others are beneficial, the goals are the most important because they helps the therapist to evaluate techniques being used and modify as such.

74. **A** This is because of the median nerve.

75. **B** Contusion is a deep bruise to the muscle. A contracture is an abnormal, and usually permanent, flexion of a joint.

76. **B** Avoid the area because it may be a hematoma. Refer client to a physician.

77. **D** Anterior pelvic tilt means the ASIS is lower than the PSIS. This means the anterior muscle attachments (rectus femoris, iliopsoas) are pulling the pelvis down in front, which indicates tightness in those muscles.

78. **C** Pectoralis major and latissiumus dorsi would not only slump the shoulders forward but would also internally rotate the arm to the point that the palms are facing the front of the thigh. Your client's palms are facing the sides of the leg like they should, so the hump forward would indicate it is a spinal curve issue.

79. **B** Chondromalacia is a condition in which the cartilage on the posterior side of the patella is worn down due to friction of the femur (usually tracking problems), and now there is bone-on-bone rubbing.

80. **D** A program that is too challenging may lead to frustration; if it is too easy, it will lead to boredom; if it is too time-consuming, they won't do any of it.

81. **D** All should be included if the referral is coming from a physician and being used for insurance reimbursement.

82. **D** The others either directly work with breathing (intercostals), or if the person is having difficulty breathing such as during an asthma attack, they begin to shoulder breathe. That would utilize the levator scapula and the upper trapezius.

83. **B** Because he is elderly it could be, worst-case scenario, related to congestive heart failure. When in doubt, refer it out.

84. **B** To relax and stretch rhomboids and erector spinae would be stretching muscles that are already stretched.

85. **A** You know it is "subjective" when you can start the sentence, "The client states . . ."

86. **C** Acute second degree sprain means there is some tearing of the ligaments. The area needs to heal first before work is done.

87. **D** Finding out how the client feels after the last massage helps the therapist determine the course of action for the next session.

88. **A** Life happens, and things don't always proceed as planned. Therefore, staying reasonably flexible will help both you and the client.

89. **B** SI joint (sacro-iliac joint) will have pain over the PSIS. The fact that she fell directly on her back is also a sign that the SI joint needs to be checked.

90. **A** Because the knee has slight rotation (the screw home mechanism), when a cartilage tear is present, the femur can catch the tear (locking feeling) or loosen from the tear (giving way). Either way, the client should see a physician.

91. **C** Think of the word "cavas" and cave; you have a cave under the foot.

92. **B** Chair techniques are not different from table massage, but the position of the client to the therapist makes facial expressions and verbal cues harder.

93. **C** Muscle guarding may give a false negative test, so you want your client relaxed when testing the injured side.

94. **D** Mental status cannot be observed best by visual observation. Also, this is factual information, not subjective.

95. **A** It's not that the second toe is longer; it's that the first toe is too short, thus causing more weight bearing on the second toe instead of the first.

96. **B** Bunions are on the side of the first toe (first metatarsal-proximal phalangeal joint); bunionettes are on the fifth metatarsal-proximal phalengeal joint.

97. **C** The transverse arch goes from the first metatarsal to the fifth metatarsal. If this falls, the toes will spread out.

98. **C** TOS has the same tingling and numbness down the arm as carpal tunnel syndrome, so sometimes people think it's carpal tunnel when it's TOS and vice versa.

99. **A** Think of the Great Plains of the Midwest; they are flat, and so are feet that have pes "planus."

100. **C** Postural asymmetry would be all right, but the answer choice states "symmetry."

chapter 5

Therapeutic Massage and Bodywork Applications

CHAPTER OUTLINE

AREAS OF COMPETENCE

This chapter includes sections that correspond to the organization of the NCBTMB exam as follows:

Therapeutic Massage Applications

NCETM (24%)

A. Theory

- Effects/benefits of massage/bodywork (physiological, emotional/psychological)

B. Methods and Techniques

- Client draping and positional support techniques
- Hydrotherapy/hydromassage application
- Stress management and relaxation techniques
- Self-care activities for the client to maintain health (e.g., stretching, swimming)
- Principles of holistic practice/approach
- Postural balancing
- Use of massage tools
- Enhancing client's kinesthetic awareness
- Joint movement techniques
- Static touch/holding
- Techniques/strokes (compression/holding/palming, cupping, flicking, friction, gliding, hair pulling, jostling, kneading, percussion, pinching, rocking, shaking, skin rolling, torquing, traction, vibration)
- Stretching (e.g., active stretching, passive stretching, resisted stretching, cross-directional stretching, proprioceptive neuromuscular facilitation [PNF], muscle energy technique [MET], reciprocal inhibition, active isolated stretching [AIS])
- Aromatherapy
- Topical analgesics
- Gauging pressure as appropriate
- Practitioner body mechanics
- Standard precautions
- CPR/first aid

NCETMB (22%)

Same as above with following additions:

- Asian energy bodywork
- Western energy bodywork

Effects of Massage

So far, we have reviewed anatomy/physiology, diseases, contraindications, indications, and how to assess our clients. Now let's take a look at massage techniques. First, we need to understand the effects of massage physiologically, emotionally, and psychologically.

Physiological Effects

- Breaks down adhesions
- Increases flexibility and mobility
- Increases joint ROM
- Balances pH levels
- Reduces chemically induced pain and inflammation
- Increases cellular metabolism
- Increases skin temperature and blood flow
- Promotes hormonal release with systemic effects
- Removes toxins and metabolic wastes
- Chemically induces vasodilation
- Improves overall blood and lymph circulation
- Hastens healing
- Improves oxygen and nutrient transfers in the body
- Affects heart rate and blood pressure
- Increases urine volume and excretion
- Facilitates sebaceous secretions
- Stretches muscles
- Improves muscle tone and relaxation
- Relieves muscle spasms, cramps, and pain
- Alleviates pain directly

- Promotes homeostasis between parasympathetic and sympathetic systems
- Promotes fluid removal from lungs (tapotement/percussion)
- Reduces stress which helps improve the immune system

Emotional Effects

- Promotes positive feelings
- Improves the connection between mind and body
- Reduces stress
- Encourages better nutrition, exercise, and health practices
- Reduces pain (physically and emotionally)
- Reduces fatigue (physically and emotionally)
- Increases productivity
- Promotes a sense of confidence and control
- Helps promote a more positive self-image

Psychological Effects

- Promotes communication and expression
- Improves self-esteem
- Improves sleep patterns
- Improves mood
- Decreases feelings of anger
- Reduces touch aversion and touch sensitivity
- Helps reduce anxiety

Methods and Techniques of Massage

Client Draping

Before the massage begins, you must appropriately drape the client. Draping is as much for the client as it is for the therapist. It serves several purposes:

1. provides a professional atmosphere
2. supports the client's need for privacy
3. offers warmth and coziness

4. allows the client to disrobe for easier access to appropriate areas for massage

Basic supine drape: The basic supine drape has the client lying on his/her back. The bolster is underneath the knees in a comfortable position, which is recommended whenever the client is in the supine position so as not to put undue pressure on the lower back. The sheet is draped on the chest so as not to expose breast tissue; this is true whether the client is female or male, in order to provide privacy. The arms can be underneath the drape or on top of the drape depending on client preference and what area the therapist is working. See Figure 5-1.

Basic anterior leg drape: This draping technique provides privacy for the client while allowing the therapist access to the thigh, leg, and foot. In Figure 5-2, the drape is pulled comfortably up to the thigh and tucked under the client for security. The rest of the sheet can be tucked under the opposite leg (as shown) or pulled under the exposed leg for what is called a "diaper drape." Either method is acceptable.

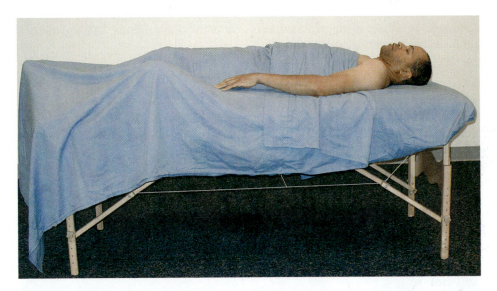

Figure 5-1 Basic supine drape.

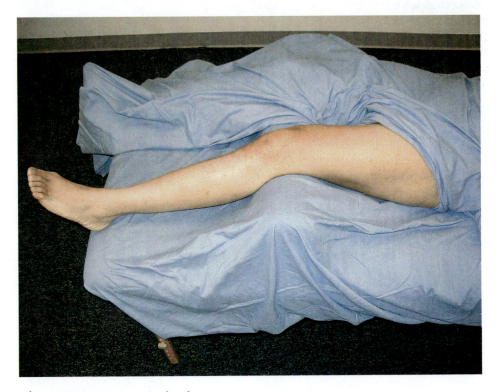

Figure 5-2 Basic anterior leg drape.

Abdominal drape: The abdominal drape allows for access to the abdominal region while maintaining privacy and comfort. A pillow case or towel is placed across the breast tissue before the sheet is pulled down below the chest. Once the pillow case is in place, the therapist can pull the sheets down to the client's waist. Tucking the sheets on the sides adds comfort. See Figure 5-3.

Prone back drape: The client is prone with the bolster underneath the ankles in a comfortable position. Placing the bolster here prevents the feet from being plantar flexed and also prevents undue pressure on the patella when massaging the legs. The sheet is pulled down to the client's waist. If the client is wearing undergarments,

the sheet should be tucked into the elastic band and on the sides for security. See Figure 5-4.

Posterior leg drape: The client is in the prone position with the bolster underneath the ankles. This draping technique is similar to the previously shown anterior leg drape in that the technique allows the therapist access to the thigh, leg, and foot. In Figure 5-5, the drape is pulled comfortably up just under the gluteals for client security. The drape can go higher if the intent is to work on the gluteals. The rest of the sheet can be tucked under the opposite leg (as shown) or pulled under the exposed leg for what is called a "diaper drape." Either method is acceptable.

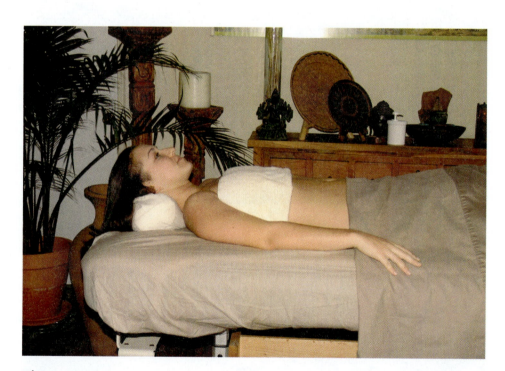

Figure 5-3 Basic abdominal drape using a towel or pillow to cover the breast tissue.

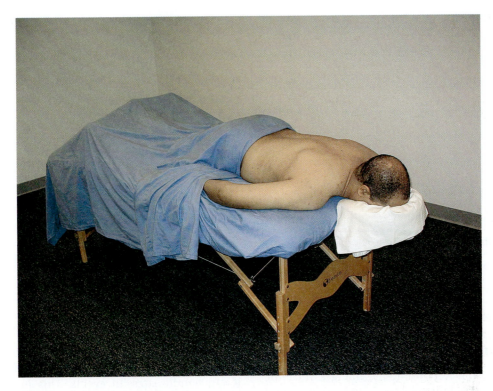

Figure 5-4 Basic prone back drape.

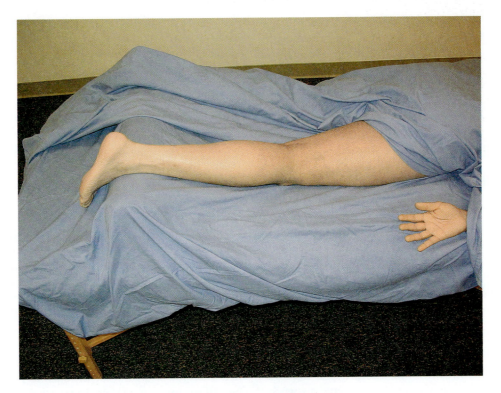

Figure 5-5 Basic posterior leg drape in prone position.

TABLE 5-1

At a Glance: Signs and Symptoms of Stress

Physical	Emotional	Behavioral
• Headaches	• Insomnia	• Alcohol or drug use
• Rapid breathing	• Depression	• Reduced sex drive
• Sweaty palms	• Anxiety	• Irritability and impatience
• Dry mouth	• Nightmares	• Anger and aggression
• Palpitations	• Crying spells	• Social isolation
• Light-headedness	• Feelings of helplessness	• Changes in appetite
• Stomach aches	• Lack of energy	• Loss of interest and boredom
• Difficulty concentrating		
• Sleep problems		

Stress Management and Relaxation

Stress is our natural response to life changes. It can be good or bad, but too much of anything is rarely a good thing. Stress manifests itself in a variety of ways. See Table 5-1 for some common signs of stress.

A variety of ways are available to help control stress. They include:

Breathing techniques: Perform deep breathing using your diaphragm, not shoulder breathing. Using your diaphragm allows more air exchange and allows the muscles to relax. Place your left hand on your chest and your right hand on your abdomen. If your right hand moves more while you breathe, you are using your diaphragm. If your left hand moves more, then you are shoulder breathing and might be stressed.

Biofeedback: Biofeedback is the ability to take information on a physiological function (such as heart rate or rate of breathing) and take control over it. For example, if you are nervous and notice you are breathing fast, you can slow down your breathing which in turn will help lower heart rate and help you relax. Or, if you are shoulder breathing, you can concentrate on using the diaphragm, thus providing a more relaxed breathing state.

Visualization: Visualization has been used by athletes for years. With this technique, you simply visualize in your mind the outcome you would like to achieve. For example, if you are nervous about giving a speech, "see" yourself in your mind giving the speech and doing it flawlessly.

Exercise: Exercise is essential for a balanced state. The stronger and more efficient the body is, the better it can handle stressful events. This includes self-care techniques for bodyworkers as well as our clients. Swimming, stretching, jogging—anything that we like to do for exercise. Prevention is the key whether it is illness or injury.

Meditation: Meditation is a deep focus that can be achieved through different means. Whether you focus on breathing, yoga, prayer, or just taking time out for yourself and relaxing, meditation is always beneficial.

Massage: The benefits of massage have been previously discussed. However, although we know the benefits, we as bodyworkers and therapists must take time to receive as well.

Other Holistic Techniques

Acupressure: This treatment is very similar to acupuncture except that acupressure requires the use of thumbs and fingertips on pressure points. These pressure points, when released, stimulate the flow of vital energy—known as "chi"—that circulates along the body's meridians and influences the functioning of some internal organs.

Applied kinesiology: In applied kinesiology, practitioners examine structural factors such as posture and gait by performing muscle tests. The practitioner applies light fingertip massage to pressure points on the body or head in order to stimulate or relax key muscles. Kinesiology is used to improve digestion, energy, and sports performance and to ease back and joint pain, allergies, asthma, depression, and headaches because we are all connected, and issues in one area can affect other areas.

Aromatherapy: Aromatherapy involves either using essential oil(s) from plants in the massage lubricant for treatment or by using these oils in candles and oil burners. Essential oils are usually blended with a carrier oil, such as jojoba or grapeseed oil. Aromatherapy is helpful in relieving a variety of symptoms including stress, sleep disorders, and anxiety, and helps enhance health and appearance. See Table 5-2 for some essential oils and their uses.

TABLE 5-2

At a Glance: Aromatherapy

Oil	Uses	Contraindications
Chamomile	Helps ease depression, stress, anger, tension, and irritability.	Not recommended for those allergic to ragweed or for those on anticoagulant medications.
Clary Sage	Antidepressant, calms, balances.	Not recommended during pregnancy or breastfeeding.
Eucalyptus	Eases respiratory congestion, brings comfort when experiencing loss and grief, and helps with mental and physical fatigue.	Use sparingly since it may irritate the skin; not recommended for children under age 2 due to possible airway spasm and cessation of breathing. Also not recommended for those with asthma, severe liver diseases or inflammatory disorders of the gastrointestinal tract or kidneys.
Juniper	Promotes sense of strength and well-being, eases muscle/joint pain.	Not recommended during pregnancy or breastfeeding, or for those with kidney disease.
Lavender	Aids in insomnia, calms and balances, helps ease irritability.	Caution must be taken if on medications that depress the central nervous system including narcotics and antianxiety or sleep medications. Consult physician.
Lemon	Energizes mind and body.	Avoid prolonged exposure to sunlight since this oil is photosensitizing; not recommended for those with high blood pressure.
Peppermint	Promotes energy and enthusiasm, eases headaches, nausea, and motion sickness.	Avoid during pregnancy and breastfeeding.
Rosemary	Stimulates mental clarity, concentration, memory.	Avoid during pregnancy or when breastfeeding; not recommended for those with epilepsy or high blood pressure.
Sandalwood	Promotes deep relaxation, abates depression, quiets the mind.	Avoid on those with kidney problems.
Tangerine	Clears away negativity, helps calm an overactive nervous system.	May cause photosensitivity.
Ylang-Ylang	Calms nervous system, eases depression, and reduces frustration.	Avoid on sensitive skin; not recommended for those with low blood pressure.

Cranio-sacral therapy (CST): CST is a gentle, hands-on method used to evaluate and enhance the functioning of the cranio-sacral system. The cranio-sacral system is comprised of the membranes and cerebrospinal fluid that surround and protect the brain and spinal cord. A soft touch is used as practitioners release restrictions in the cranio-sacral system to improve the functioning of the central nervous system.

Deep connective tissue massage: This deep form of bodywork helps to release myofascial restrictions in the body. Chronic tension, range of motion, posture, and self-awareness can all be improved with deep connective tissue massage because it restores length and flexibility to the fascia, normalizing the tissue and bringing greater circulation to the fascia.

Deep tissue massage is commonly used interchangeably with 'Clinical Massage' and with 'Deep pressure massage.' The primary techniques used in deep tissue massage are ischemic compression, cross-fiber friction, myofascial release, flushing effleurage, and joint mobilization and stretching. The first step is to assess the injury by reviewing the client intake form, postural assessments, joint range of motion, etc. The second step is to prepare the area by applying lubricant and warming up the areas with effleurage and pretrissage techniques. The next phase is the palpatory phase where tissues are explored for abnormalities or pathologies. The fourth phase is the treatment phase where the aforementioned techniques of ischemic compression, cross-fiber friction, myofascial release, flushing effleurage, and joint mobilization and stretching are used. The interval phase is where the therapist moves to another treatment area in order to give this area time to rest. Then the therapist will retreat the area and hopefully find less pain and tension. The recovery phase is where the tissues are flushed with a final treatment of effleurage to help remove metabolic waste and reduce soreness. The aftercare phase is the last phase where the therapist instructs the client concerning the use of ice, proper hydration, stretches, and any modifications in his/her activities of daily living (ADLs).

Hydrotherapy: Hydrotherapy involves the use of water, in any form, in massage therapy. This technique is often incorporated with other types of therapy previously listed. It has indications and contraindications that must be followed (see Table 5-3).

Hot stone therapy: Stones of all shapes and sizes and varying temperatures, ranging from 130–140 degrees F, are used during stone massage therapy to elicit physical healing, mental relaxation, and a spiritual connection to earth energy. Warm stones encourage the exchange of blood and lymph and provide soothing heat for deep-tissue work. Cold stones aid with inflammation, moving blood out of the area. Stones are placed in varying positions on the body. The alternating heat and cold of thermotherapy helps vasoconstriction and vasodilation to allow the exchange of oxygen and waste products in the body.

Integrative manual therapy: A combination of structural and functional rehabilitation, integrative manual therapy has roots in osteopathic medicine. Its basic concept is that no parts of the body function independently—it is all connected. If structure is affected, function is affected and in turn, other areas become affected. Manual therapy addresses the entire body, locating the source of pain and disability, not just the symptoms.

Manual lymph drainage: Manual lymph drainage (MLD) is a very gentle therapy that works to improve functioning of the lymphatic (immune) system. Recall from Chapter 1 that lymph is very thick and hard to move. Muscle contractions help it to circulate through the body, but lymphatic drainage can help the process along further. Light pressure is used because the lymph vessels are located just under the skin. The therapy cannot be done through sheets since direct contact with the skin is necessary. No oil or lubricant is used.

TABLE 5-3

At a Glance: Hydrotherapy

	Heat	Cold
General Uses	• Promote circulation of blood and lymph • Relieve cramps and muscle spasms • Relieve stress (mental and physical)	• Reduce inflammation and secondary injury • Relieve pain • Relieve muscle spasms • Promote healing
Local Effects	• Surface vasodilation and redness • Increase in leukocyte migration through cell walls • Muscle relaxation • Increase in local swelling • Increase in cell metabolism • Local analgesia	• Initial vasoconstriction • Decrease in circulation • Decrease in leukocyte migration through cell walls • Decrease in cell metabolism • Muscle contraction • Numbing, analgesic effect
Systemic Effects	• Increase in heart rate • Increase in nervous system stimulation, then sedation • Increase in digestive process • Decrease in cellular metabolism internally	• Increase in nervous system stimulation, then sedation • Initial increase in heart rate, then decrease • Increase in cellular metabolism
Contraindications	• Inflammation • Circulatory/heart conditions • Pregnancy • Geriatric client • Infant • Cancer • Impaired nerve sensitivity	• Circulatory/heart conditions • Pregnancy • Geriatric client • Infant • Cancer • Impaired nerve sensitivity

Muscle energy technique: A technique that when applied directly is based on the principle of reciprocal inhibition and when applied indirectly is based on post-contraction relaxation. The goal is to relax muscle spasms.

Myofascial release: This slow and subtle technique can be used to release fascia and muscle throughout the body. The therapist uses light to moderate traction and a twisting approach to achieve a relaxation of the fascia and improve circulation.

Neuromuscular therapy: This therapy is applied with a combination of effleurage or gliding, petrissage or grasping, friction, muscle energy, and strain/counter-strain techniques. The goal is the release of trigger points and to improve circulation. It also helps in re-alignment of posture by relaxing hypertonic tissue.

On-site chair massage: This takes place when a massage therapist goes to the client, whether it is in the client's home or at the workplace. The client is clothed for the treatment. Some employers hire massage therapists to perform 10–15-minute massages at the workplace or at events to promote a practice.

Perinatal massage: Many methods of massage are effective and safe prenatally, during labor, and postpartum. Specific techniques can reduce pregnancy discomfort and enhance the physiological and emotional well-being of both mother and fetus. During labor, skilled, appropriate touch facilitates and shortens the process while easing pain and anxiety. In the postpartum period, specialized techniques rebalance structure, physiology, and emotions of the new mother. Infant massage may help her to bond with and care for her infant. Pregnant women should ask their doctor if massage is recommended, as many massage therapists require a physician's referral. The massage therapist will have specialized, advanced training in anatomy, physiology, complications, precautions, and contraindications.

Reflexology: Reflexology is an ancient healing art based on the principles that there are reflexes or zones in the hands and feet that correspond to every part, organ, and gland in the body. By using acupressure and massage on the hands and feet, the client benefits from improved circulation, detoxification, reduced tension, and the body's ability to heal itself.

Shiatsu therapy: Developed in Japan, shiatsu is a finger-pressure technique utilizing the traditional acupuncture points. Similar to acupressure, shiatsu concentrates on unblocking the flow of life energy and restoring balance in the meridians and organs in order to promote self-healing. With the client reclining, the practitioner applies pressure with the finger, thumb, palm, elbow, or knee to along the energy meridians. Benefits may include pain relief and a strengthening of the body's resistance to disease and disorder.

Sports massage: Sports massage consists of specific components designed to reduce injuries, such as alleviating inflammation and providing a warm-up for amateur and professional athletes before, during, after, and within their training regimens. Massage can help an athlete prepare for a competitive event. A pre-event massage is brief and invigorating, usually lasting 15–20 minutes. It is given within an hour before the sporting event through the clothes. Post-event massage will be calming and relaxing with the goal of easing pain and soreness and reducing inflammation, also lasting 15–20 minutes and through the clothes. Post-event massage can bring blood and oxygen to tense areas and flush out metabolic waste products built up during heavy muscle use.

Swedish massage: One of the most commonly taught and well-known massage techniques, Swedish massage is a vigorous system of treatment designed to energize the body by stimulating circulation. Five basic strokes flow toward the heart to improve circulation and elimination of waste as well as a variety of other benefits as discussed in Chapter 5. Therapists use a combination of kneading, rolling, vibration, percussive and tapping movements, with the application of oil to reduce friction on the skin.

Thai massage: Thai massage is based on the theory that the body is made up of 72,000 *sen*, or energy lines, of which 10 hold top priority. Thai massage involves peripheral stimulation, meaning it acts as an external stimulant to produce specific internal effects. This point serves as the main division between Thai and Western massage. Thai massage is practiced on a firm mat on the floor instead of on a table, instrumental in the effective use of the practitioner's body weight. Except for the feet, the client remains fully clothed, so draping is not necessary.

Massage Techniques and Strokes

The following section presents the various massage strokes and techniques you will need to know to pass the exams—and to provide great client care! See Table 5-4. You will also learn how to judge pressure and depth, how to stretch, and how to maintain good body mechanics.

Holding: Holding allows for quiet focus for both client and therapist (Figure 5-6). It allows the client to adjust to being touched and to begin the relaxation process. Incorporated with deep breathing, compression lets the client fall deeper into relaxation. It can be used at the beginning or end of a massage.

Compression: Compression is pressure into the body to help spread the tissue.

TABLE 5-4

At a Glance: The Basic Massage Strokes

Stroke	Purpose
Holding	Allows for quiet focus for both client and therapist; allows the client to adjust to being touched and begin the relaxation process. Generally used as the initial or resting position.
Compression	Pressure into the body to help spread tissue against underlying structures.
Effleurage	Helps to warm up the muscles, spread the lubricant, and let the client adjust to your touch; also known as gliding.
Petrissage	Helps to work deeper tissues, therefore is generally done after effleurage; also known as kneading.
Friction	Breaks down adhesions.
Vibration	Enhances relaxation, increases circulation, relieves pain, relieves upper respiratory tract congestion, and reduces trigger and tender point activity.
Tapotement	Stimulates nerve endings, helps with decongesting the lungs, tones atrophied muscles, increases local blood flow, and relieves pain.

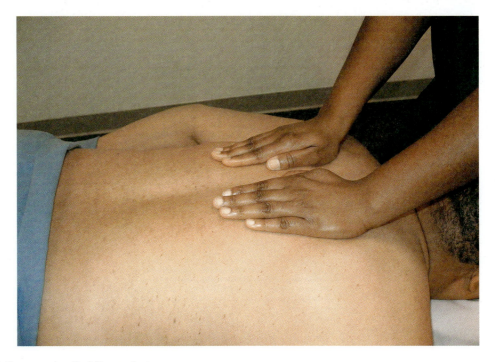

Figure 5-6 Compression/holding technique.

Effleurage: Effleurage helps to warm up the muscles, spread lubricant, and let the client adjust to your touch; it is also known as gliding (Figure 5-7).

It is usually one of the first strokes used on the client and is excellent for assessing and exploring tissues, calming the nervous system when done slowly, stimulating the nervous system when done quickly (such as sports massage), soothing areas, and relaxing the client. Various techniques of effleurage include raking, ironing, circular, and nerve stroke.

Petrissage: Petrissage helps to work deeper tissues, and is therefore generally done after effleurage; it is also known as kneading (Figure 5-8). The tissues are grasped and lifted so the underlying tissue can be wrung, kneaded, or squeezed. This stroke increases blood flow, works out metabolic waste, reduces local swelling, relaxes and lengthens muscle tissue, softens superficial fascia, releases endorphins, and relieves general fatigue. Techniques include skin rolling, praying hands, and ocean waves.

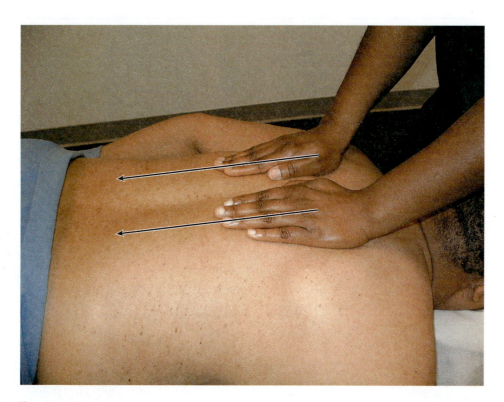

Figure 5-7 Effleurage technique.

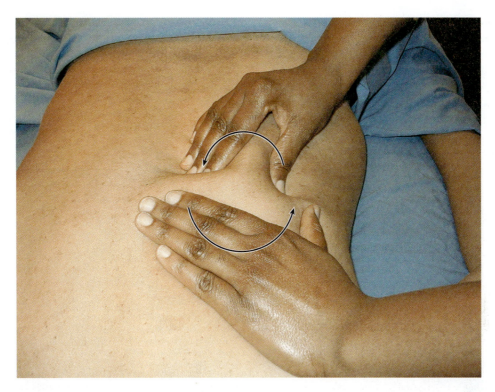

Figure 5-8 Two handed petrissage.

Friction: Friction combines compression and movement. It breaks down adhesions and is generally done after effleurage and petrissage to ensure proper warm-up of muscles (Figure 5-9). Other benefits of friction include generating heat, dilating capillaries, loosening stiff joints, promoting and increasing circulation, and reducing trigger point formation. Techniques include cross-fiber, circular, parallel, chucking, wringing, and rolling.

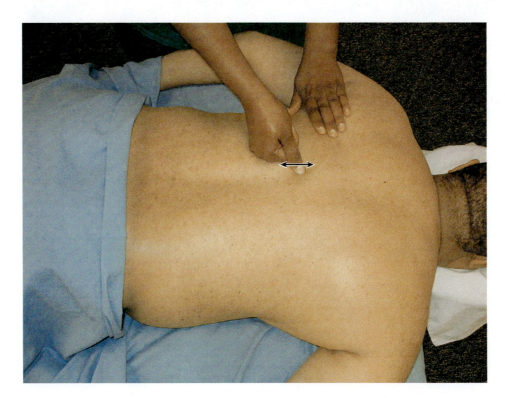

Figure 5-9 Friction technique.

Vibration: Vibration is a rapid shaking, quivering, or trembling technique (Figure 5-10). Benefits include enhancement of relaxation, increasing circulation, relief of pain, relief from upper respiratory tract congestion, and reduction in trigger and tender point activity. Variations include jostling, rocking, and fine vibration.

Tapotement: Tapotement is also known as percussion and utilizes striking movements. Benefits include stimulating nerve endings, decongesting the lungs, toning atrophied muscles, increasing local blood flow, and relieving pain. Various techniques include slapping, tapping, pulsing, raindrops, pinching, hacking, cupping, pounding, clapping, and diffused. See Figures 5-11 through 5-14.

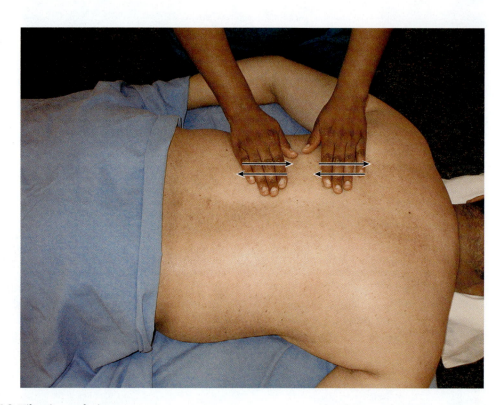

Figure 5-10 Vibration technique.

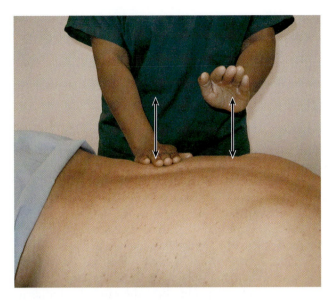

Figure 5-11 Slapping tapotement.

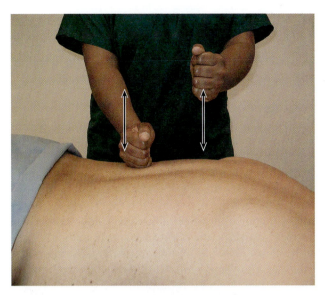

Figure 5-13 Pounding tapotement.

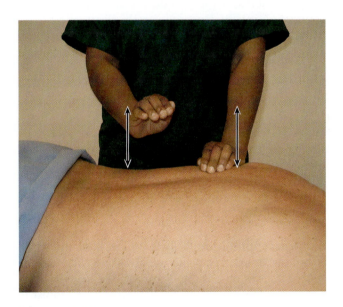

Figure 5-12 Cupping tapotement.

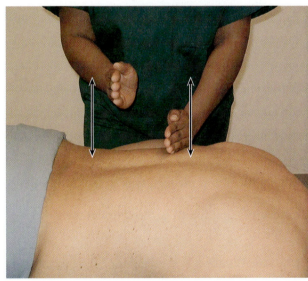

Figure 5-14 Hacking tapotement.

Judging Pressure and Depth

Judging pressure and depth is important in order to work the muscles as needed without harming the client and/or the muscle tissues and other structures.

Pressure: Pressure can be achieved by using various body parts including hands, elbows, knuckles, palms, and forearms. Various tools are made that allow the therapist to apply pressure (for example, T-bars and knobs). Clients often affect how much pressure can be applied. Letting the client know he or she is allowed to say whether the pressure is too much or too little is the best course of action although it does not always happen. Watching the client's facial expressions, if possible, helps. Also, tuning into muscular tension, guarding, and changes in breathing will let the therapist know if the pressure is too much.

Depth: This is how far into the tissues the therapist can go. Several factors influence this:

- purpose or intent of the massage stroke
- condition of the tissue
- the type of stroke the therapist is using
- area of the body where pressure is applied
- response of the client

Excursion: Excursion is the length of the stroke and how far it has traveled.

Speed: Speed is how fast or slowly the strokes are applied.

Rhythm: Rhythm is the regularity of the strokes.

Continuity: Continuity is the uninterrupted flow of strokes.

Duration: Duration is the length of time spent on a particular area of the client.

Stretching Techniques

Active stretching: Active stretching occurs when the client does his/her own stretching, and one muscle contracts to stretch the opposing muscle. For example, while the client is lying supine on the floor, he/she activates his/her quadricep muscles to lift his/her leg in the air in order to stretch the hamstrings.

Passive stretching: Passive stretching occurs when the therapist lifts the client's limb in order to stretch a

muscle, and both agonist and antagonistic muscles are relaxed. Using the same example as above, the therapist lifts the client's leg and pushes it back until the client says to stop or the therapist feels resistance. The client does not have to activate any muscles because the therapist is doing the work.

Proprioceptive neuromuscular facilitation (PNF): PNF stimulates neural proprioceptors to help muscles stretch farther than they normally would. Using the same hamstring example as above, the therapist takes the client's leg back as far as first resistance is felt (passive). Then the client is asked to contract the hamstrings/gluteals by pushing his/her leg against the therapist (active). This activates the Golgi tendons. This isometric contraction is generally held for six to eight seconds. When the client relaxes, the Golgi tendons can completely relax and allow the muscle spindles to take over. This allows the therapist to push the client's leg back farther. If the client is very tight, repeat two to four times. Disadvantages are (1) if the client has heart problems or high blood pressure, the isometric contraction is very dangerous on the heart, and (2) by using close to 100 percent resistance, both the client and therapist risk getting hurt. However, advantages are that (1) clients can stretch farther than they normally would be able to stretch, and (2) it allows for strengthening of the muscle(s).

Muscle energy techniques (METs): METs are very similar to PNF with one exception—the client only uses about twenty percent resistance on the contraction phase. This decreases the risk to the therapist and/or client for injuries and is safe to use with high blood pressure and heart patients.

Reciprocal inhibition: This is an excellent stretching technique to use for acute muscle cramps as well as general stretching; it is also known as Sherrington's law. Reciprocol inhibition ensures that when the agonist is moving or activated, the antagonist elongates. For example, using the same hamstring stretch to relax a cramp in the hamstrings, the quadriceps group is contracted isometrically. Maintain the contraction for ten to twenty seconds, then release. Repeat three to four times.

Active isolation stretching (AIS): This is another technique that can be used for general stretching that follows the Sherrington law. It is often used as a warm-up to activity in order to make stretching more functional rather than for cramping situations like reciprocal inhibition. In other words, why perform static stretches sitting or standing still to prepare for activity that requires movement? This is an excellent technique for sports massage pre-event. Let's look at a quadriceps stretch: the client activates the hamstrings to flex the knee and stretch the quads. The client keeps lifting the heel to the buttocks trying to get the heel closer and closer to the buttocks. This stretches the quads farther and farther. Repeat this about ten times, holding each only for about one second. On the tenth repetition, grasp the ankle and hold the quadriceps stretch. Repeat on the other leg.

Practitioner Body Mechanics

As stated in Chapter 4, the effects of gravity can help or hinder a massage therapist/body worker. Pressure should come from the therapist's legs if proper mechanics are used. Table height, along with thickness of the client and treatment techniques, also plays a role.

Proper alignment: When the therapist is in proper position, the ears should line up with the shoulders; the shoulders should line up with the greater trochanter; the knee of the front leg should not go beyond the toes; and body weight should be primar-

ily on the heel of the foot when pressure is applied. If the knee travels in front of the toes, body weight is on the ball of the foot, and pressure is on the knees, leading to future problems. With the weight on the heels of the feet, and knees behind the toes, the body weight is more on the quadriceps muscle group. The two main stances are the bow stance, or lunge (Figure 5-15), and the warrior stance, or horse stance (Figure 5-16).

Bow stance/lunge: As shown in Figure 5-15, you can see the shoulder-hip-knee alignment. The knee does not shift anteriorly in front of the toes on the front leg. This is an excellent stance for strokes such as effleurage, compression, holding, and friction.

Warrior stance/horse stance: This stance, as shown in Figure 5-16, is an excellent stance to use during petrissage. The therapist is facing the client from the side. Both knees are bent and the shoulder-hip-knee alignment is apparent. The toes are slightly turned outward in order to take stress off the knees when the therapist shifts his/her body weight for the petrissage. The knees, once again, do not travel in front of the toes.

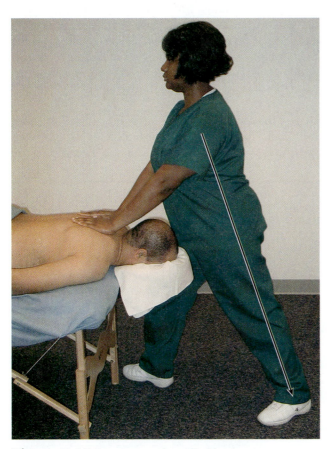

Figure 5-15 Bow stance, also called lunge.

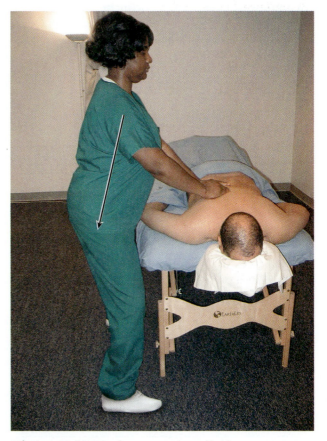

Figure 5-16 Warrior stance, also called horse stance.

Standard Precautions and Procedures

Bloodborne pathogen rule: The bloodborne pathogen rule should be followed by all health care professionals. It essentially states that one should assume that we all have some communicable condition. When dealing with body fluids, we should protect ourselves appropriately by using latex (or latex-free, if allergic) gloves and cleaning our equipment, tables, and paraffin baths. The importance of washing hands cannot be overstated. Although HIV/AIDS is transmissible via body fluids, Hepatitis B can live outside of the body for up to seven days. Therefore, protect yourself and protect your client.

Cardiopulmonary resuscitation (CPR): All massage therapists and bodyworkers must maintain their CPR certifications. See Tables 5-5 and 5-6 for a review of basic CPR and choking procedures following American Heart Association guidelines.

First aid: The need for first aid can come in a variety of situations and can occur at any time. Generally, environmental issues might occur at sports massage events. Fractures may also occur at these events. Quick and immediate care is imperative as is contacting the medical tent or calling 9-1-1.

Hyperthermia

Hyperthermia: Hyperthermia can be caused by a combination of the following environmental and physi-ological factors. One of these must exist in order for symptoms to manifest:

1. Hot AND humid weather
2. Dehydration due to profuse sweating coupled with a lack of proper fluid intake
3. Electrolyte imbalances (e.g., sodium, potassium, and magnesium)
4. Hypoglycemia due to insufficient or improper food intake prior to event
5. Insufficient cardiovascular conditioning for hot weather competition
6. Inordinately long competition (e.g., triathlon, marathon)

Risk factors may include older adults due to loss of muscle mass, exercise and exertion, obesity, heavy clothing, certain drugs (alcohol, amphetamines, diuretics, beta blockers), hyperthyroidism, infection/fever, poor acclimatization, and cardiovascular disease.

Pathological Stages of Heat Illness/Injury

Heat cramps: Heat cramps are due to fluid/electrolyte imbalances resulting from excessive dumping of fluids without replacement. *Symptoms*: profuse sweating and muscle cramps with normal body temperature. *Treatment*: increase fluid intake (water, electrolyte drink) and massage cramp. If symptoms do not improve within a few minutes, treat as heat exhaustion.

Heat exhaustion: Heat exhaustion is the most common heat illness occurring with athletes because they generally "work through" the cramps. Because of the

TABLE 5-5

At a Glance: CPR			
	Adult (age 8 and up)	Child (1–8 years)	Infant (0–1 years)
Rescue Breathing (person has a pulse) Number of breaths	1 breath every 5 seconds (10–12 breaths per min) 1:5	1 breath every 3 seconds (20 breaths per min) 1:3	1 breath every 3 seconds (20 breaths per min) 1:3
CPR: Rate of compressions	100/min	100/min	100/min
Depth of Compression	$1\frac{1}{2}$–2 inches	$\frac{1}{3}$–$\frac{1}{2}$ inches	$\frac{1}{3}$–$\frac{1}{2}$ inches
Ratio	30 compressions/ 2 breaths 30:2	30 compressions/ 2 breaths 30:2	30 compressions/ 2 breaths 30:2
Hand Position	2 handed	1 handed	2 fingers
Pulse Location	Carotid pulse	Carotid pulse	Brachial pulse

TABLE 5-6

At a Glance: Choking

Adults and Children over 1 Year Conscious Victim	Babies and Infants	Unconscious Victim or When Rescuer Can't Reach Around Victim
Someone who cannot answer by speaking and can only nod the head has a complete airway obstruction and needs emergency help.		
Determine if the person can speak or cough. If not, proceed to the next step.	Determine if the infant can cry or cough. If not, proceed to next step.	Place the victim on back. Facing the victim, kneel astride the victim's hips. With one of your hands on top of the other, place the heel of your bottom hand on the upper abdomen below the rib cage and above the navel. Use your body weight to press into the victim's upper abdomen with a quick upward thrust. Repeat until object is expelled. If the victim has not recovered, proceed with CPR. The victim should see a physician immediately after rescue.
Perform an abdominal thrust (Heimlich maneuver) repeatedly until the foreign body is expelled.	Give 5 back blows.	
A chest thrust may be used for markedly obese persons or women in late stages of pregnancy.	Give 5 chest thrusts.	
If the adult or child becomes unresponsive, perform CPR; if you see an object in the throat or mouth, remove it.	Repeat steps 2 and 3 above until effective or the infant becomes unconscious. If the infant becomes unresponsive, perform CPR; if you see an object in the throat or mouth, remove it.	

continued dumping of body fluids, a cardiovascular condition called hypovolemia begins to manifest (hypo = low; volemia = volume; "low blood volume"). *Symptoms:* profuse sweating, normal or high body temperature, dilated pupils, early fatigue, headaches, nausea, confusion, cold-clammy skin, weakness, decreased coordination, hypotension (BP lower than 90 for the systolic—a concern because this is after they have been exercising when it would normally be higher), strong rapid pulse, and finally collapse.

Treatment: move victim to a cool place to reduce further sweating and fluid loss; call paramedics if BP is lower than 90 for the systolic pressure. If victim is conscious and BP is 90 to 100 for systolic, attempt to give fluids; however, intravenous fluids would be best. Victim should avoid activity for at least twenty-four hours and should drink adequate amounts of fluids during that time. The victim should refrain from exercising in the heat for at least one week because he/she is especially susceptible to repeat episodes within that period.

Heat stroke: Heat stroke is less common than heat exhaustion, but it is more serious. Heat stroke results from the body's inability to dissipate heat. This is a true medical emergency. In order to protect the heart and brain from the side effects of hypovolemia, the body overrides the cooling system by shutting down the sweating process. This returns cardiac filling, core blood pressure, plasma volume, and venous blood flow to normal. Unfortunately, the outside temperature is so high, the body temperature continues to rise, and the body literally begins to cook itself from the inside out. *Symptoms*: the three classic symptoms are (1) high body temperature (106 degrees F or higher), altered consciousness, and lack of sweating—the classic hot, dry skin. However, dry skin is not always reliable since the victim may be wet with previous sweat from exercising. This heat illness can result in death. *Treatment*: call 9-1-1 and the event first aid tent immediately. Until help arrives, get client to a cool place indoors or in the shade if outside. Place cold, wet towels on pulse points, but watch for shivering (you do not want the victim to go into shock). If the client begins to shiver, remove cold towels and only use cool sponging. Heat stroke causes permanent damage to the thermoregulatory system, and individuals who have experienced it should not exercise in hot humid environments any more since they will always be susceptible to this life-threatening situation.

Hypothermia

Hypothermia: Hypothermia can be caused by a combination of cooler temperatures, being scantily clad, lower heat production, dehydration, inexperience (the athlete who runs the second half of a race slower than the first half, lowering the body's heat production, and causing sweat from the first half of the race to create chills). *Symptoms:* include dehydration, hypotension, shivering, euphoria, slurred speech, dilated pupils, edema of the face, cloudy consciousness, low body temperatures, increased muscle tonus, intoxicated appearance, and pale skin.

Pathological stages of hypothermia: (1) Slow breathing, (2) collapse, and (3) death. Symptoms can progress very rapidly.

Fractures: Again, this is not typically seen in a massage office environment; however, if you are at a sports massage event, this might occur. There are several types of fractures as noted in Table 5-7. The best first aid is to stabilize the client and call the medical tent and/or 9-1-1.

TABLE 5-7

At a Glance: Fractures	
Simple fracture	The bone is broken but does not protrude through the skin. Also known as a closed fracture.
Compound fracture	The bone is broken and DOES protrude through the skin. Also known as an open fracture.
Stress fracture	A small hairline fracture in a bone usually caused by prolonged repetitive activity.
Compression fracture	An impacted fracture characterized by crushed bones.
Comminuted fracture	A fracture in which three or more bone fragments are produced. Also known as shattered.
Greenstick fracture	An incomplete fracture, more common in children.

*Some questions are not directly addressed in this chapter, but are meant to act as a general review of subjects studied in various school curriculums.

Questions

Therapeutic Massage Applications
NCETM (24%) NCETMB (22%)

1. The type of heat illness that is a medical emergency is
   A. heat cramps.
   B. hypothermia.
   C. heat stroke.
   D. heat exhaustion.

2. Symptoms of hypothermia include all of the following EXCEPT
   A. decreased muscle tonus.
   B. slurred speech.
   C. edema of the face.
   D. dehydration.

3. The bloodborne pathogen rule states that
   A. not everyone has a transmittable disease, so take precautions when necessary.
   B. gloves are only needed when dealing with body fluids.
   C. precautions are less for body workers.
   D. treat everyone (including yourself) as if they might have a communicable condition.

4. Safety has two aspects for the massage therapist; safety of the massage facility and
   A. safety of the procedure performed.
   B. safety of the office equipment.
   C. handicap accessibility.
   D. fire codes.

5. For the massage therapist to provide safe procedure, he/she must be trained in human physiology, pathophysiology, first aid, CPR, and
   A. NMT.
   B. sports massage.
   C. endangerment sites.
   D. driver's license.

6. Hand washing for the therapist should include
   A. washing of hands.
   B. washing of nails.
   C. washing of forearms.
   D. All of the above are correct.

7. Which of the following is not recommended for the massage therapist to wear because it is difficult to remove microorganisms from them?
   A. ornate rings
   B. bracelets
   C. watches
   D. All of the above are correct.

8. Which statement is true concerning HIV-positive clients?
   A. broken skin or cuts are not a concern since they do not have AIDS
   B. massage will not help them at all
   C. the risk is too high to massage them
   D. None of the above are correct.

9. The three worst substances to use on your table and accessory vinyl are
   A. soap, water, and oil.
   B. soap, alcohol, and chlorine bleach.
   C. oils, alcohol, and chlorine bleach.
   D. oils, vinegar, and soap.

10. Disinfect your massage table
    A. after each client.
    B. when it comes in contact with body fluids.
    C. once a week.
    D. once a month.

11. After giving abdominal thrusts to an unconscious adult for obstructed airway, your next step is to
    A. give two slow breaths.
    B. check for the object in mouth.
    C. retilt the head.
    D. check for pulse.

12. What is the combination of water, friction, soap, or other disinfecting agents to eliminate the presence of microorganisms called?
    A. aseptic techniques
    B. diseptic techniques
    C. unhealthy
    D. sterilization

13. When giving rescue breaths, which should you do if you do not suspect a neck injury?
    A. lift the chin
    B. head tilt
    C. head tilt and chin lift
    D. lift head with hand behind the neck

14. What is the first step in a basic emergency?
    A. call 9-1-1
    B. check the scene
    C. assess the victim
    D. ABC's

15. Abdominal thrusts help a choking victim by
    A. forcing air in the lungs out through the airway to push an object out.
    B. using the pressure forced on the abdominal muscles to force the air out.
    C. pushing on the stomach in order to use gas to push the object out.
    D. All of the above are correct.

16. Chemical packs are used for
    A. pain relief and relaxation of muscle spasm.
    B. mild sprained ankle.
    C. treating an injury using a cooling effect.
    D. All of the above are correct.

17. Contrast baths
    A. are effective after seventy-two hours of a new injury.
    B. help to pump out waste products through alternating vasoconstriction and vasodialation.
    C. always begin and end with ice.
    D. All of the above are correct.

18. Surfaces that come in direct contact with the client during hydrotherapy treatments as well as all reservoirs that collect perspiration or exfoliated skin cells must be cleaned
    A. after each treatment.
    B. at the end of the day.
    C. once a week.
    D. once a month.

19. Nail care includes keeping nails clean and
    A. short and neatly trimmed.
    B. polished.
    C. short and ingrown.
    D. long and neatly trimmed.

20. Which is best applied to a first degree burn?
    A. cool water
    B. warm water
    C. ointment
    D. dry bandage

21. Your client is at your office and is having slight chest pain radiating to his jaw, but he denies it is a heart attack. He tells you in absolute terms not to call 9-1-1. You should
    A. respect your client's wish, send him home, and call him that evening to make sure he is OK.
    B. go ahead and do the massage since it might be a trigger point.
    C. call 9-1-1 immediately.
    D. None of the above are correct.

22. Your client has no pulse but is breathing. You should
    A. give chest compressions.
    B. call 9-1-1.
    C. begin CPR.
    D. recheck the pulse.

23. Which of the following is the first step when initiating CPR?
    A. assess for open airway
    B. palpate carotid pulse
    C. position the person on his/her side
    D. place hands below xiphoid to begin chest compressions

24. What should you do for the conscious adult who appears to be choking but can cough a little?
    A. give an abdominal thrust
    B. lower the person to the floor and open the airway
    C. call 9-1-1 immediately
    D. nothing

25. The one type of environmental condition that people cannot acclimatize to is
    A. altitude.
    B. humidity.
    C. heat.
    D. cold.

26. Your client comes to you with a severely bruised ankle with swelling from mid lower leg to the toes. What may have happened?
    A.   1st degree sprain
    B.   2nd degree strain
    C.   3rd degree sprain
    D.   3rd degree strain

27. The number one source of microorganism cross-contamination is by
    A.   unclean massage linens.
    B.   hand to hand contact.
    C.   toilet seats.
    D.   sneezing.

28. Your athlete just sprained his/her ankle. The order of actions you should take for treatment would be
    A.   rest, ice, compression, elevation.
    B.   rest, ice, compression, evacuate.
    C.   movement, ice, compression, elevate.
    D.   look, listen, feel.

29. Universal precautions may include which of the following?
    A.   mandatory hand washing
    B.   the use of cotton gloves
    C.   using unclean massage sheets
    D.   All of the above are correct.

30. How long should you massage your soapy hands and forearms when washing them?
    A.   ten seconds
    B.   thirty seconds
    C.   forty-five seconds
    D.   one minute

31. To properly clean underneath the nails, use a/an
    A.   nail file.
    B.   nail brush.
    C.   orange stick.
    D.   Both B and C are correct.

32. The client may refuse the massage for sanitation reasons if
    A.   you have an open wound.
    B.   you have an infection.
    C.   you have a dark mole on your hand.
    D.   Both A and B are correct.

33. What is the process of removal of pathogenic micro-organisms by a chemical or mechanical agent?
    A.   sterilization
    B.   hygiene
    C.   disinfection
    D.   septic techniques

34. If there is any blood or tissue fluid seepage due to any superficial wounds, remove the linens with gloved hands and wash in
    A.   hot water.
    B.   hot water, detergent, and chlorine bleach.
    C.   hot water and chlorine bleach.
    D.   hot water, detergent, and ammonia.

35. Which one of the following is not important in providing a safe, germ-free, and barrier-free environment for the practice of massage therapy?
    A.   safe and unobstructed passage
    B.   hydraulic massage table
    C.   fire extinguisher
    D.   lever style door handles

36. The universal sign for choking is
    A.   coughing.
    B.   grasping the throat.
    C.   waving the hand.
    D.   All of the above are correct.

37. An athlete comes to you during an event. He just sprained his ankle. You should
    A.   perform light effleurage to reduce the risk of swelling.
    B.   refer him to the first aid tent.
    C.   put ice on it.
    D.   tell him it's nothing and send him on his way.

38. Which type of burn is more characterized by blistering but no tissue necrosis?
    A.   first degree
    B.   second degree
    C.   third degree
    D.   fourth degree

39. Handwashing is important
    A.   after each massage session.
    B.   only if the client is dirty.
    C.   before and after each massage session.
    D.   it does not matter.

40. The type of heat illness generally characterized by hot dry skin is
    A.   heat cramps.
    B.   heat stroke.
    C.   heat exhaustion.
    D.   Both B and C are correct.

41. When massaging a woman with large breasts or breast implants
    A. give her a rolled-up towel or cylindrical pillow to be placed under or above the breasts
    B. perform side-lying massage only
    C. do not adjust your normal massage positioning
    D. None of the above are correct.

42. Which one of the following is not appropriate when confronted with an emotional release of crying by a client?
    A. leave the room immediately to give them privacy
    B. approach the emotional release with acceptance
    C. remind your client that tears are OK
    D. ask the client if they would like for the massage to continue

43. When working with a visually impaired client, you should not
    A. announce your presence in a loud voice.
    B. orient them to their surroundings.
    C. tell them what you are going to do and what you would like for them to do.
    D. begin the massage until after they know you are in the room.

44. METs stands for
    A. muscle elongation techniques.
    B. muscle energy techniques.
    C. movement elongation techniques.
    D. movement energy techniques.

45. Cryotherapy refers to the application of
    A. heat.
    B. water.
    C. ice.
    D. liniments.

46. Cryotherapy is
    A. not beneficial to cramps.
    B. a technique that should not be used on bruises.
    C. is not beneficial in hypothermia.
    D. can be used on Raynaud's disease.

47. Friction is best used to
    A. increase the CNS.
    B. decrease the parasympathetic nervous system.
    C. decrease scar tissue and adhesions.
    D. Both A and B are correct.

48. Static stretching is defined as
    A. gently stretching a muscle until resistance is met and holding it for ten to twenty seconds.
    B. stretching a muscle one inch into the resistance and then holding it for a short period of time.
    C. stretching in which a bounce or bobbing forces tissue to release.
    D. vigorously stretching with the aid of another person.

49. Local application of cold for acute pain, sprains, and trauma provides a/an
    A. anticoagulant effect.
    B. numbing, analgesic effect.
    C. protective, inflammatory effect.
    D. consensual, reflexive effect.

50. When performing METs, the client pushes against the therapist using how much force?
    A. ten percent
    B. twenty percent
    C. forty percent
    D. close to 100 percent

51. When performing METs, the therapist holds the stretch for _____, then the client relaxes for _____.
    A. two seconds, eight seconds
    B. ten to fifteen seconds, ten to fifteen seconds
    C. eight seconds, two seconds
    D. it doesn't really matter

52. METs are useful for all of the following EXCEPT
    A. warming up tissues.
    B. strengthening weakened tissues.
    C. immobilizing articulations.
    D. reducing swelling and edema.

53. What strokes are good for bronchitis?
    A. petrissage
    B. effleurage
    C. tapotement
    D. friction

54. The client with bursitis in his or her shoulder should
    A. receive a massage on that shoulder.
    B. utilize ice on the affected shoulder.
    C. receive NMT on the subscapularis, supraspinatus, infraspinatus, and teres.
    D. utilize heat on the affected shoulder.

55. Proper positioning for postural drainage for sinuses is
    A. client is supine with head above the body.
    B. client is supine with feet above the body.
    C. client is prone with head above the body.
    D. Both B and C are correct.

56. The percussion technique includes
    A. hacking.
    B. petrissage.
    C. rocking.
    D. friction.

57. The technique that is generally used to spread the massage lotion/cream is
    A. petrissage.
    B. friction.
    C. tapotement.
    D. effleurage.

58. What is a physiological effect of hydrotherapy?
    A. rejuvenation and rehabilitation
    B. vasodilatation and vasoconstriction
    C. burning, tingling, numbing
    D. manual lymphatic drainage

59. The application of cryotherapy can be done by
    A. hot packs.
    B. steam bath.
    C. ice bucket.
    D. compresses.

60. In order to help promote joint flexibility, the best stroke to use is
    A. vibration.
    B. rocking.
    C. friction.
    D. tapotement.

61. The primary benefit of deep transverse friction is to
    A. loosen joints.
    B. improve circulation of blood.
    C. improve circulation of lymph.
    D. break up adhesions and scar tissue.

62. The technique that involves lifting, grasping, rolling, and compressing muscles is
    A. effleurage.
    B. tapotement.
    C. kneading.
    D. friction.

63. The way that cryotherapy reduces swelling is by
    A. vasoconstriction.
    B. vasodilatation.
    C. release of endorphins.
    D. hyperemia.

64. What technique might be beneficial for a client who is over her chest cold, but still has congestion in the chest?
    A. petrissage
    B. friction
    C. tapotement
    D. effleurage

65. What is the most common physiological effect of Swedish massage?
    A. increased blood flow
    B. decreased mental stress
    C. feeling of more energy throughout the day
    D. clearer mind and thought process

66. Which technique involves strokes to break up adhesions in the tendons?
    A. Cyriax
    B. petrissage
    C. general friction
    D. tapotement

67. Muscle energy techniques utilizes what method in this form of stretching?
    A. ballistic stretching
    B. passive stretching
    C. active stretching
    D. isometric contraction with resistance

68. PNF and MET are very similar methods of stretching; however, there are differences. What is (are) the difference(s)?
    A. MET requires the client exert to 100 percent of his or her strength in the resistance phase
    B. PNF is not as safe to use on those with high blood pressure
    C. MET does not have an isometric resistance phase
    D. PNF can only be used on athletes

69. The shaking technique is a type of
    A. percussion.
    B. tapotement.
    C. vibration.
    D. hacking.

70. Which of the following techniques would benefit an amputee when massaging the stump?
    A. friction
    B. effleurage
    C. petrissage
    D. tapotement

71. Effleurage strokes should be applied by
    A. using vigorous movements.
    B. smooth movements towards the heart.
    C. smooth movements away from the heart.
    D. counterclockwise, circular movements.

72. The best technique for the asthmatic client is
    A. deep, relaxing strokes.
    B. vigorous and stimulating strokes.
    C. none, because massage is contraindicated.
    D. superficial and relaxing strokes.

73. The type of technique that is effective in toning the muscles is
    A. tapotement.
    B. petrissage.
    C. effleurage.
    D. vibration.

74. Kneading is accomplished by
    A. sliding the hands rapidly over the skin.
    B. lifting, grasping, rolling, and compressing the muscles.
    C. locating an adhesion and rapidly massaging over it.
    D. tapping the fingertips on the surface of the skin.

75. Which of the following statements is true regarding precautions for pregnant women?
    A. do not lay the client on her back for long periods of time
    B. contraindications are the same as for a non-pregnant client
    C. do not use effleurage on the abdomen
    D. All of the above are true.

76. The technique you are using requires firm pressure, but your client states it is causing pain. What should you do?
    A. stop the massage
    B. stop the technique
    C. tell them "no pain, no gain"
    D. back off on the pressure and continue communication with the client

77. When addressing pressure with the client during the massage, it is helpful to
    A. ask the client to simply raise a hand if pain is felt.
    B. use the one to five point scale where one is no pain and five is excruciating pain.
    C. ask the client to stand as much discomfort as possible, especially when doing deep tissue work.
    D. Both A and B are correct.

78. The two most basic foot stances a therapist uses during massage are the
    A. L stance and bow stance.
    B. bow stance and horse stance.
    C. anatomical position and bow stance.
    D. None of the above are correct.

79. When applying massage therapy, it is often best to work
    A. from specific to general.
    B. the area of complaint only.
    C. from general to specific, then general again.
    D. only the areas the therapist feels needs attention.

80. Which of the following are used when applying massage strokes?
    A. intention, pressure
    B. rhythm and continuity
    C. speed and duration
    D. All of the above are correct.

81. Which of the following consists of a cycle of rhythmic lifting of the muscle tissues away from the bone or underlying structures with the hollow of the palms, followed by firmly kneading or squeezing the muscle with a gentle pull toward the therapist ending with a release of the tissue?
    A. effleurage
    B. petrissage
    C. friction
    D. tapotement

82. When applying pressure, it is important to
    A. not exceed the client's personal pain threshold.
    B. cause muscle relaxation.
    C. take into consideration the area on the body where the pressure is being applied.
    D. All of the above are correct.

83. In sports massage, maintenance massage is
    A. quick and brisk.
    B. light and general.
    C. a blend of soreness reduction and specific work.
    D. trigger point massage.

84. Given appropriate therapy and client compliance, grades one and two lesions usually heal in about
    A. four to eight weeks.
    B. twenty-four to seventy-two hours.
    C. six months.
    D. not until all trigger points and spasms are diminished.

85. An excellent stroke for assessing tissues is
    A. effleurage.
    B. petrissage.
    C. friction.
    D. percussion.

Answers and Explanations

Therapeutic Massage Applications
NCETM (24%) NCETMB (22%)

1. C   Heat stroke occurs when the thermoregulatory system has shut down. Body temperature can rise to very dangerous levels and cause permanent brain damage and even death.

2. A   When an individual is so cold that he/she goes into hypothermia, the muscles tend to tense up; therefore, muscle tonus increases.

3. D   Because the client may not be aware that he/she has something transmittable, bodyworkers and other healthcare workers should always use precautions to protect themselves and to protect clients.

4. A   All are important, but the question asks about safety FOR the massage therapist.

5. C   Endangerment sites is the best answer because massaging over these sites can place the client at risk. Remember—do no harm.

6. D   Because we use other techniques that use the forearms, it is necessary to clean the forearms as well.

7. D   This is due to the fact that skin cells, bacteria, and other contaminants can get into the jewelry and be spread from client to client.

8. D   As many of us know now, HIV can be transmitted through body fluids, so latex gloves should be worn if the therapist or client has HIV and one of them has an open cut or wound. The benefits of massaging an HIV-positive client are basically the benefits of anyone. The reduction of stress in itself is beneficial.

9. C   Alcohol and bleach will dry out and crack the vinyl of your table or chair. Also, if it is not completely wiped off and your client comes into contact with it, it can irritate his/her skin, nose, eyes, and other mucous membranes.

10. A   Tables should be disinfected after each client. Although the linens and mattress pads might protect the table somewhat, body fluids can still reach the massage table.

11. B   If there is an object where you can reach with pincher fingers, you might be able to get it out.

The step after checking for the object is two full breaths.

12. A   "Septic" or "sepsis" means contaminated. Add the "a" which means "away from," and this now means "from contaminated." Sterilization takes a very detailed process and is not accomplished by hand washing.

13. C   This is an effective and safe way to open the airway if there is no suspicion of a neck injury. If a neck injury is suspected, you should do the jaw thrust in order to stabilize the neck.

14. B   Check the scene to ensure safety for you and for the victim.

15. A   The abdominal thrusts are forcefully pushing on the diaphragm to force out air and, hopefully, the object blocking the airway.

16. D   Chemical packs provide a cooling effect. Although ice may be best, it can still be used on a mild ankle sprain.

17. D   Because heat is involved, contrast baths should not be used on new injuries. Because of the analgesic effect and vasoconstriction of the ice, it is best done first and last in the entire treatment.

18. A   This is general practice of hygiene.

19. A   Nail polish can hide dirty nails; ingrown nails can get infected; and long nails, as studies have shown with healthcare workers in hospitals, can transmit disease by microorganisms getting caught under the free edge of the nail.

20. C   This will help the skin heal since it is a superficial burn.

21. C   With symptoms like this, the first sign that he might be having a heart attack is that he denies that he is having a heart attack. Many people think they will be embarrassed if you call 9-1-1, but your best bet is to call 9-1-1 and let the client argue with the EMTs as to whether he/she goes to the ER. From a liability standpoint and out of concern for your client, you've done your job.

22. D   Recheck the pulse since it is impossible for someone to be breathing with no pulse. Now, someone can have a pulse and not be breathing, and in that case, call 9-1-1 and begin rescue breathing. But the scenario given here is not possible.

23. A   The ABC's are Airway, Breathing, and Circulation.

24. D Because the person can cough, air is getting in and out; therefore, he/she might be able to cough up the object. If you try to attempt something, you may lodge the object farther down and completely block the airway. So, stand by, keep an eye on him/her, and let him/her cough.

25. D This is why Eskimos still wear coats!

26. C With the swelling and discoloration, your client probably completely tore ligaments as well as the joint capsule. The synovial fluid leaking out would cause all the swelling.

27. B Our hands touch so many things and people that they can become very contaminated. Hand washing is the best way to reduce your risks of coming in contact with something. Studies have actually shown that toilet seats can be very clean because people avoid sitting on them out of concern for contamination.

28. A This is the RICE principle.

29. A Cotton gloves are porous and will allow bacteria and other material onto the hands or the surface being touched. As massage therapists, we always maintain clean, washed linens.

30. B You should wash for at least thirty seconds in order to utilize the frictioning to clean better.

31. D These will help clean out material under the nail close to the nail bed.

32. D A dark mole may be malignant, but is not a risk for the client.

33. C Sterilization uses heat, water, chemicals, and gases—a much more involved technique than what is listed in this question.

34. B The detergent and chlorine bleach will help disinfect and clean. The hot water will also help kill germs.

35. B The others listed are safety devices; the hydraulic table is more of a luxury device rather than a safety device.

36. B When someone is choking, they generally grasp the throat to show they are choking.

37. C The FIRST thing is to put ice on it; the second thing is to get him to the first aid tent.

38. B First degree generally causes superficial redness of the skin (for example, hot water). Second degree causes blistering (a bad sunburn), and third degree is the life-threatening type due to tissue death (necrosis).

39. C This is self-explanatory—good hygiene is important.

40. B Generally, hot dry skin is related to heat stroke because the thermoregulatory system has shut down and the body is unable to sweat. In some circumstances, keep in mind if the individual has been exercising, the skin may feel damp from sweat they excreted prior to the heat disorder.

41. A This will help make lying prone a little more comfortable.

42. A A therapist should never leave the room during a massage unless the client requests it.

43. A They are visually impaired, not hearing impaired.

44. B METs are Muscle Energy Techniques—a type of permanent elongation stretch.

45. C Cryotherapy is the application of ice or cold.

46. C Cryotherapy (the use of ice) is very beneficial to cramps and bruises to decrease the spasm effect and to decrease blood flow. Raynaud's disease is a peripheral circulatory and vascular disorder. Putting ice on affected areas will decrease blood flow even more and may cause the skin to turn bluish. "C" is the answer because you don't want to put ice on someone who is already cold.

47. C Friction decreases the central nervous system, and it increases the parasympathetic nervous system. The general purpose of friction is to reduce or realign scar tissue and adhesions to assist with increase of range of motion.

48. A Static stretching involves finding a comfortable position and holding the stretch for at least ten seconds without bouncing so as to activate the muscle spindles and deactivate the Golgi tendons; this is in order to assist the muscle in relaxation efforts for lengthening.

49. B Ice is not a blood thinner nor is it a blood thickener, so "A" is not the answer. "C" isn't right because ice does not cause inflammation; it helps to decrease it. "D" doesn't work well because your body and your emotions do not work consensually to vasoconstrict the blood vessels. Therefore, "B" is the best answer; ice numbs, and because it numbs, it is analgesic.

50. B This is the advantage of METs over PNF, making it safer on client and therapist.

51. C This is standard practice in METs; this allows for the Golgi tendons to completely relax so the muscles spindles can take over and allow for more ROM during the stretch.

52. C METs is a form of stretching; we don't want to immobilize, we want to mobilize tissue.

53. C The thumping action of tapotement will help loosen phlegm.

54. B Ice should be used to treat inflammation, which is what bursitis is. There is not a whole lot a therapist can do in a bursitis situation except let it heal, and then work on the muscular issue. A light massage may be done, but the best answer here is "B."

55. A Elevating the head above the lungs helps with drainage—especially sinus drainage. If the client is prone, placing the head below the body will help, unless he or she has high blood pressure. In that case, it should not be done prone due to the excess stress on the blood vessels of the brain.

56. A Petrissage is a form of kneading; rocking is a type of vibration; and friction is friction.

57. D With the long glides of effleurage, this helps to warm the muscles up and to spread the lotion.

58. B This question is asking for the physiological. "A" and "C" deal with personal, subjective views. Manual lymphatic drainage is another type of modality but is not an effect of cryotherapy

59. C Cryotherapy involves ice. The other choices involve heat.

60. C Friction helps break up adhesions that can act as glue to the tissue and limit range of motion.

61. D Friction helps break up adhesions that can act as glue to the tissue and limit range of motion.

62. C Tapotement is thumping or percussion-type strokes; friction is a brisk compression-type stroke; and effleurage is a smooth, gliding stroke.

63. A Cryotherapy means ice therapy. Ice constricts the blood vessels and helps restrict or prevent more metabolic waste from getting to the injured site to lessen swelling.

64. C The thumping of tapotement would be beneficial to help loosen any phlegm that may still be in the chest. Since the client is over the cold, the risk of passing it to the therapist is low. If a concern exists, a mask can be worn.

65. A Increased blood flow is the only answer choice dealing with physiological changes. The others are more psychological changes and effects.

66. A While general friction and kneading help break up adhesions in the belly of the muscle,

Cyriax—a technique created by James Cyriax—helps break up adhesions in the tendon.

67. D This is because METs have an active phase where the therapist positions the body part to be stretched (passive stretching), and the client has a resistance phase where he/she pushes against the therapist (active stretching). If "both B and C" were available, that would be correct, but since it is not, "D" is the correct answer.

68. B Because PNF stretching utilizes 100 percent (or close to it) resistance from the client, those with high blood pressure should not perform PNF stretching. Isometric contractions with a higher exertion can cause the blood pressure to go up even higher, especially in those individuals who already have high blood pressure. Therefore, the twenty percent or so resistance used in METs would be better and safer.

69. C Vibration enhances relaxation, increases circulation, relieves pain, relieves upper respiratory tract congestion, and reduces trigger and tender point activity. Tapotement (which includes percussion and hacking) stimulates nerve endings, helps with decongesting the lungs, tones atrophied muscles, increases local blood flow, and relieves pain.

70. D Tapotement would be best to help increase circulation.

71. B Effleurage strokes also help spread the cream/lotion, and warm up the muscles for other techniques.

72. D Deep strokes may be too invigorating thus causing a "stressor" and aggravating an asthmatic attack or response.

73. A This is because tapotement causes the muscles to contract and then relax.

74. B Kneading is also known as petrissage. "A" describes effleurage done quickly; "C" describes friction; and "D" describes tapotement.

75. A First of all, as the pregnancy progresses, lying flat on the back will be uncomfortable. Placing pillows appropriately while the client is on her back is recommended. Even still, lying on the back for long periods of time can cause the baby to sit on the mother's vena cava and cause light-headedness.

76. D It is not necessarily the technique but the pressure, so decrease the pressure and make sure the client is comfortable.

77. D "No pain, no gain" is not true. If too much pain is felt, the muscles will respond by tightening up more, which is not what you want.

78. B   The bow stance is like a lunge and the horse stance is standing with feet apart facing the table/client and leaning side to side. This is useful for petrissage strokes.

79. C   Remember that if a client has a particular area of pain, there are probably other muscles affected outside of the pain zone. Work generally first to help warm up the muscles.

80. D   Intention, pressure, speed, duration, rhythm, and continuity are all important when applying massage strokes.

81. B   Tapotement is thumping or percussion-type strokes; friction is a brisk compression-type stroke; and effleurage is a smooth, gliding stroke.

82. D   Not exceeding the client's personal pain threshold is important because if it is exceeded, the client will tense and muscle guard, hindering the relaxation process. The muscle relaxation process is important physically and mentally. Taking into consideration the area on the body where the pressure is being applied is also important because lighter pressure is needed over bony landmarks, and endangerment sites need to be considered.

83. C   Because athletes may hurt after a hard day of training, it helps to reduce muscle soreness to prepare them for the next day of training.

84. D   When dealing with injuries, it is very hard to give time frames. Each person heals differently.

85. A   Effleurage strokes also help spread the cream/lotion and warm up the muscles for other techniques, but because they are nice long strokes, the therapist can take note of hypertonicities, lumps, etc.

chapter 6

Professional Standards, Ethics, Business, and Legal Practices

AREAS OF COMPETENCE

This chapter includes sections that correspond to the organization of the NCBTMB exam as follows:

NCETM (6%) NCETMB (6%)

A. Maintaining professional boundaries while responding to client's emotional needs
B. Client interviewing techniques
C. Communication with other health professionals
D. When to refer clients to other health professionals
E. Verbal and non-verbal communication skills
F. NCBTMB Code of Ethics and Standards of Practice
G. Issues of confidentiality
H. Legal and ethical parameters of scope of practice
I. Basic psychological and physical dynamics of practitioner/client relationships
J. Planning strategies for single and multiple sessions
K. Session record-keeping practices
L. Basic business and accounting practices
M. Outsourcing business needs (e.g., insurance billing, bookkeeping)
N. Regulations pertaining to income reporting
O. Need for liability insurance
P. State and local credentialing requirements
Q. Legal entities (e.g., independent contractor, employee)

Strategies to Success

Manage your time!

It's easy to develop good study habits if you manage your time effectively. Every day, set aside a time when you can study without interruption. Don't let anything else intrude on this time—not shopping, not paying bills, not running errands, not socializing with friends, not even family (unless it is a true emergency). In this way, you will have study time and will still be able to get everything else done. Write a daily to-do list, including study time, and check tasks off as you complete them.

Professionalism is a must, and this includes understanding legal and ethical parameters. How you speak, what you say, and how you present yourself all tell clients and other health-care professionals about your professionalism. Legitimacy and qualifications should always be truthful. When in doubt, refer it out. Your character is what you are willing to do if no one can see you and no one will ever find out. Your ethics are your morals and principles. Your integrity is your wholeness and honesty. Your image is you and who you are.

The NCBTMB Code of Ethics provides guidelines for practice.

The NCBTMB Code of Ethics

The Code of Ethics of the National Certification Board for Therapeutic Massage and Bodywork (NCBTMB) requires certificants to uphold professional standards that allow for the proper discharge of their responsibilities to those served, that protect the integrity of the profession, and that safeguard the interest of the individual clients.

Massage and bodywork therapists shall act in a manner that justifies public trust and confidence, enhances the reputation of the profession, and safeguards the interest of individual clients. To this end, massage and bodywork therapists in the exercise of accountability will:

I.   Have a sincere commitment to provide the highest quality of care to those who seek their professional services.

II. Represent their qualifications honestly, including education and professional affiliations, and provide only those services that they are qualified to perform.

III. Accurately inform clients, other health-care practitioners, and the public of the scope and limitations of their discipline.

IV. Acknowledge the limitations of and contraindications for massage and bodywork and refer clients to appropriate health professionals.

V.   Provide treatment only where there is reasonable expectation that it will be advantageous to the client.

VI. Consistently maintain and improve professional knowledge and competence, striving for professional excellence through regular assessment of personal and professional strengths and weaknesses and through continued education and training.

VII. Conduct their business and professional activities with honesty and integrity, and respect the inherent worth of all persons.

VIII. Refuse to unjustly discriminate against clients or other health professionals.

IX. Safeguard the confidentiality of all client information, unless disclosure is required by law or necessary for the protection of the public.

X. Respect the client's right to treatment with informed and voluntary consent. The certified practitioner will obtain and record the informed consent of the client, or client's advocate, before providing treatment. This consent may be written or verbal.

XI. Respect the client's right to refuse, modify, or terminate treatment regardless of prior consent given.

XII. Provide draping and treatment in a way that ensures the safety, comfort, and privacy of the client.

XIII. Exercise the right to refuse to treat any person or part of the body for just and reasonable cause.

XIV. Refrain, under all circumstances, from initiating or engaging in any sexual conduct, sexual activities, or sexualizing behavior involving a client, even if the client attempts to sexualize the relationship.

XV. Avoid any interest, activity, or influence which might be in conflict with the practitioners' obligation to act in the best interests of the client or the profession.

XVI. Respect the client's boundaries with regard to privacy, disclosure, exposure, emotional expression, beliefs, and the client's reasonable expectations of professional behavior. Practitioners will respect the client's autonomy.

XVII. Refuse any gifts or benefits intended to influence a referral, decision, or treatment that are purely for personal gain and not for the good of the client.

XVIII. Follow all policies, procedures, guidelines, regulations, codes, and requirements promulgated by the National Certification Board for Therapeutic Massage and Bodywork.

Permission to reprint by the NCBTMB.

In order to maintain your NCBTMB certification, the therapist must earn 50 CEC's every 4 years. Two (2) of those 50 CEC's must be on Roles and Boundaries, and four (4) must be Business/Ethics related.

Professional Considerations

Interviewing techniques: Intake forms are a must. These forms provide information about the client's health and assist in determining if medical clearance is needed prior to the massage or whether modifications are necessary. Being a good listener and observer and having the ability to ask the right questions, as well as open-ended questions, are also necessary to complete a successful interview.

Communication techniques: There are positive techniques and negative techniques when it comes to communication. Positive techniques can be used to help a client realize he or she is improving or can improve. Oftentimes, we use negative techniques to communi-cate late payments or cancellations. This is where we need to be careful to get our points across, but handle the situations appropriately. Mirroring our clients can be beneficial. If our clients are whispering, obviously they do not want others to hear; therefore, we whisper. However, if our clients are yelling, we do not want to mirror them. Other communication techniques include empathy (the ability to put yourself in another person's shoes), non-judgment, concern, and genuineness.

Table 6-1 reviews some verbal skills we can use to let our clients know we are listening and hearing what they are saying.

Nonverbal skills can also be positive or negative. Positive nonverbal communication can include a head nod, leaning in to show interest, a friendly wave, a smile, or a handshake with good eye contact (Figures 6-1 and 6-2). Negative nonverbal communication includes fidgeting, foot tapping, frowning, and lack of eye contact.

TABLE 6-1

At a Glance: Verbal Skills

Technique	Definition
Paraphrasing	Restating what the client said in order to confirm understanding.
Summarizing	Consolidating all the statements the client has said to confirm understanding.
Minimal encouragers	These are brief words such as "aha" or "I see" that let your client feel you are listening and encouraging him or her to continue.
Probing	This is an attempt to gain more information. Statements such as "Let's talk about that" will help reveal more information.
Clarifying	This is an attempt to understand what the client is saying. Such statements can include "I'm confused about what you said about your symptoms."
Confronting	This provides the client with mild or strong feedback about what is really going on, such as when dealing with a cancellation. A positive way of starting off could be, "It seems to me you have several irons in the fire. Let's work together to figure out the best course of action to help you feel better."

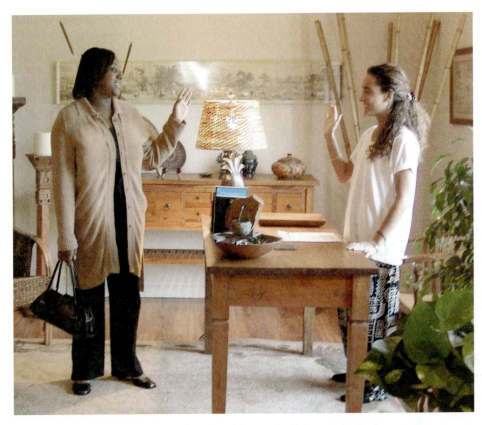

Figure 6-1 A friendly wave and smile are examples of positive nonverbal communication.

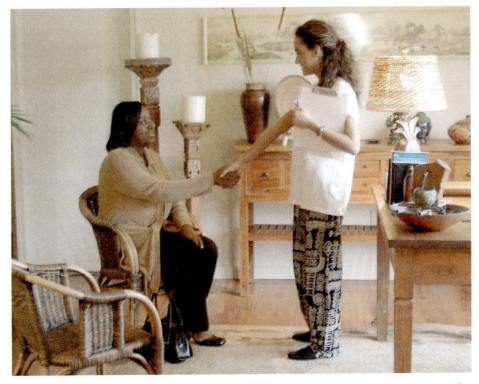

Figure 6-2 Another exmple of positive communication is offering a handshake while maintaining good eye contact.

Record Keeping

Confidentiality is of utmost importance—in fact, it's the law. Even when working out of your home, client files must be kept secure and locked. SOAP notes are the general record-keeping format in the medical profession. The following explains the SOAP note format:

S: **Subjective**: If the statement can start with, "Client states . . ." then it goes in the subjective section.

O: **Objective**: This includes what the therapist feels through palpation and sees through postural analysis, gait analysis, and range of motion tests. Changes noted by the therapist from the massage session can also be noted here. Only facts are stated in the objective section, not assumptions.

A: **Assessment/Application**: This is what the therapist did. What stretches did you do? What muscles did you focus on? What techniques and strokes did you use? What areas did you not work and why? If your client came back to you in six months and said, "Do what you did last time," you could do it because it would be noted in this section.

P: **Plan/Progression**: This is where you note suggestions to your client, for example, to see a physician or other health-care professional if necessary, stretches to do at home (how often, hold how long), when to come back, water intake, Epsom salt baths, and so on.

HIPPA stands for Health Insurance Portability and Privacy Act. The goal is to ensure that an individual's health information is protected while allowing the appropriate health care professional access to promote the highest quality of health care and to protect the public's well being. It was enacted August 21, 1996. The privacy rule applies to all health plans, health care clearing houses, and health care providers (which of course, includes massage therapists). The privacy rule protects all "individually identifiable health information whether it's by media, electronically transmitted, written, or oral (www.hhs.gov)". Individually identifiable health information, including demographic data, includes the individual's past, present, or future physical or mental health condition; the provision of health care to the individual; or past, present, or future payment for the provision of health care to the individual. "A major purpose of the Privacy Rule is to define and limit the circumstances in which an individual's protected health information may be used or disclosed by covered entities. A covered entity may not use or disclose protected health information, except either: (1) as the Privacy Rule permits or requires; or (2) as the individual who is the subject of the information (or the individual's personal representative) authorizes in writing." (www.hhs.gov). In order for information to be disclosed to another individual or business, the client must provide written consent for the specific information to the specific individual/company. This also includes any information on the client for a directory to which others may have access. Also, health care providers cannot give any information to family or friends of the client unless the client has provided in writing that it is approved to do so. This includes leaving phone messages with any identifiable characteristics. Other ways to protect client's privacy are:

- By speaking quietly when discussing a patient's condition with family members in a waiting room or other public area;
- By avoiding using patients' names in public hallways and elevators, and posting signs to remind employees to protect patient confidentiality;
- By isolating or locking file cabinets or records rooms; or by providing additional security such as passwords on computers maintaining personal information.

Planning Single and Multiple Sessions

Several considerations must be taken into account when planning single and multiple sessions.

- **Current condition**—First and foremost, consider the current condition of the client. Is it curable? Is it in my scope of work? Do I need a referral? How serious is it?
- **Goals**—These depend on the client as well as the therapist. How dedicated is the client to do what is recommended by the therapist? What the client is able to do oftentimes sets the course of action the therapist takes. How well the client releases and relaxes during the session also plays a role in future goals and sessions.
- **Effort of the client and therapist**—This could include stretches before, during, and after the session, home treatments, and equipment the therapist has available (e.g., hydroculators).

- **Frequency of sessions**—This will depend on client time and money and time and appointment availability of the therapist.
- **Contraindications**—Contraindications are set forth by the therapist or other healthcare professional but also by the client him/herself.
- **Referrals**—The necessity of referrals can sometimes delay treatment, although it is important and necessary, and they also may limit the types of therapy that can be provided, if at all.

Business Concepts

Contractor versus employee: The Internal Revenue Service (IRS) has very strict standards as to what makes an employee or a contractor. See Table 6-2 for highlights of contractor versus employee status. Whether these are pros or cons for the therapist is an individual choice.

TABLE 6-2

At a Glance: Contractor or Employee

Contractor

- sets own hours (unless more than one therapist uses the same room)
- can work for competitors
- has control over fees
- is paid per client/task/project
- must pay self-employment taxes
- purchases own supplies (although it is tax deductible)
- uses own vehicles (which has tax deductible aspects)
- must pay for recertification, continuing education, CPR recertification, and other professional licensure (which are tax deductible)
- must purchase liability insurance, health insurance, general liability insurance
- receives no payment for sick days, vacation

Employee

- cannot work for the company competitors
- has a set schedule
- is paid hourly
- company must offer benefits such as health insurance, vacation, sick days
- company can offer to cover costs for continuing education, CPR recertification
- may use company car, if available
- falls under company liability insurance and general liability insurance
- company provides basic supplies

Types of Business Entities

Sole proprietorship: In a sole proprietorship, you are in business for yourself, but you do not incorporate, create a partnership, or form Limited Liability Corporation (LLC). Your social security number is generally your company identification number. However, you can get an Employer Identification Number (EIN) if you plan to have employees. Advantages and considerations are noted in Table 6-3.

Partnerships: This type of business entity is where two or more people contribute assets, share expenses, and operate together as the business. Table 6-4 reviews advantages and considerations.

TABLE 6-3

At a Glance: Advantages and Considerations to Sole Proprietorship

Advantages	Considerations
It is easy to set up.	You are a contractor with your own company.
You have possession of profits.	You pay self-employment taxes and quarterly/annual income taxes.
You have control of all decisions.	You file a Schedule C with your 1040 form.
You have simple financial record keeping.	Your liability is increased in that if you are sued, your personal assets can be a part of the claim and reward.

TABLE 6-4

At a Glance: Advantages and Considerations to Partnership

Advantages	Considerations
Government regulations are still fairly minimal.	You can be held personally responsible for debts and legal issues, even if made without your consent.
Financial record keeping is not as complicated as a corporation.	
You have an FIN (Federal Identification Number).	
Each partner submits a copy of a K-1 report to report his/her share of profits or losses on their individual tax returns.	

S-Corporation: This is a business entity that is separate from the owner as an individual. Owners are considered employees of the business and are paid as employees. Table 6-5 reviews advantages and considerations to this business entity.

Licenses, permits, and registrations: These can vary from state to state; see Table 6-6 for a review of basic licenses, permits, and regulations.

TABLE 6-5

At a Glance: Advantages and Considerations to S-Corporation

Advantages	Considerations
You and your personal assets are separate from the business and its assets.	It is complicated to structure and generally requires an attorney to incorporate.
The business can continue if an owner leaves or dies.	You will need stock certificates, shareholders, meetings, officers.
You have a reduction in the potential for double taxation.	Return form 1120-S must be filed annually.
It allows owners/shareholders to directly declare business losses on their individual tax returns.	

TABLE 6-6

At a Glance: Licenses, Permits, and Registrations

Provisional license	Some states that have licensure for massage therapists and bodyworkers will give you a provisional or temporary license pending passing of the state licensure exam. Specifics on requirements for this license vary from state to state.
Occupational license	This license allows any business to operate.
Sales tax permit	This is required if you plan to sell any product to a client.
Registration of business name	You must be registered with the city, county, or parish office where your business will be conducted. This is your business name (other than your own name).

Insurance Needs

All massage therapists and bodyworkers and their businesses need different types of insurance. It protects you, your business, and your client.

Professional liability: Also known as malpractice insurance, this covers liability costs if you are accused of negligence. Negligence is failure to do what you should have done or doing something you should not have done that causes harm. For massage therapists and bodyworkers, this is generally dealing with soft tissue damage or damage done during the massage session itself. The importance of having professional liability insurance cannot be overstated. Whether you are guilty or not, you will still have expenses to cover, and this is where the role of insurance is important.

General liability: This covers trips, falls, property damage to your client, and personal injury when your client is on your premises. This would include if a lightpost on your property fell and hit your client's car or if your client stumbled and fell on the steps to your office entrance.

Business personal property: This covers fixed business office supplies such as your table, desk, and stereo equipment.

Health insurance: This covers you, the therapist, and your health. Major medical covers hospital stays only.

Disability insurance: This is also for you, the therapist, in case you are unable to work. Short-term disability is a temporary situation. Long-term disability can be permanent.

Accounting Terms

Granted, we did not get into this field to become accountants. However, the need to know basic accounting terms is important. See Table 6-7 for basic terminology.

TABLE 6-7

At a Glance: Accounting Terms

Term	Definition
Accounts payable	Money you owe to other vendors
Accounts receivable	Money owed to you by other vendors
Assets	Things that provide value to the company, such as massage tables, equipment, and furniture
Cash flow	The amount of money going into and out of the company
Depreciation	The process of spreading out the deduction of the cost of an asset over time
Gross income	All the money earned or accumulated before deductions
Inventory	Unsold retail items on hand
Net income	Gross income minus expenses and after taxes

Strategies to Success

Test-Taking Skills

Eliminate wrong answers!

When answering multiple-choice questions, you can increase your chances of answering correctly by eliminating answers you know are wrong. As you read the possible answers, put an X next to the ones you know are incorrect or cross them out completely. Once you have narrowed down your possible choices, you have a better chance of making an educated guess about the correct answer.

*Some questions are not directly addressed in this chapter, but are meant to act as a general review of subjects studied in various school curriculums.

Questions

Professional Standards, Ethics, and Business and Legal Practices
NCETM (6%) NCETMB (6%)

1. How many CEC's does one need to receive and in what time frame in order to maintain the NCBTMB and NCETM certifications?
   A. 50 CEC's in four years
   B. 50 CEC's in five years
   C. 50 CEC's in two years
   D. 50 CEC's in three years

2. A typical session termination procedure would include
   A. notifying the client of the session termination.
   B. asking the client to leave the premises, re-establishing therapist safety.
   C. documenting the session termination in writing in an incident report.
   D. All of the above are correct.

3. The ideal massage room temperature is between
   A. sixty to seventy degrees.
   B. seventy to eighty degrees.
   C. seventy-eight to eighty-five degrees.
   D. sixty-eight to seventy-five degrees.

4. Which of the following is a contraindication during pregnancy unless massage is ordered by the physician?
   A. weight gain
   B. Braxton-Hicks contractions
   C. edema
   D. eclampsia

5. Often including principles for therapeutic relationships, professional behavior, and business policies, which of the following is a set of guiding moral principles that influence one's course of conduct?
   A. code of ethics
   B. scope of work
   C. patient's bill of rights
   D. HIPAA law

6. The certification process for massage therapists usually involves
   A. completion of required number of hours of classroom time.
   B. apprenticeship and/or internship.
   C. successful passing of exams covering science and applied skills.
   D. All of the above are correct.

7. Non-disclosure of privileged information is called
   A. integrity.
   B. communication.
   C. confidentiality.
   D. transference.

8. Pricing of services is influenced by which of the following?
   A. location
   B. types of services
   C. overhead
   D. All of the above are correct.

9. Which of the following is NOT an allowable deduction for income tax purposes?
   A. depreciation of equipment
   B. supplies for the office
   C. revenue
   D. utilities

10. The voluntary process of completing training in knowledge and skill by a non-governmental institution such as a trade school is called
    A. certification.
    B. registration.
    C. accreditation.
    D. licensure.

11. Which of the following should NOT be included in an incident report?
    A. date, time, and exact location of the occurrence
    B. who was present at the reported incident
    C. the social security number of the client
    D. what was done to alleviate the problem at the time of the incident

12. You share office space with another therapist but operate independently. This means that
    A. because you share space you must file joint taxes.
    B. you should incorporate separately and maintain separate accounts.
    C. you should file separately only if you both earn more than $1000.
    D. None of the above are correct.

13. As an independent contractor, you must submit your taxes
    A. as quarterly estimated taxes.
    B. as bi-annual estimated taxes.
    C. as you would your personal taxes.
    D. not at all if you accept cash only.

14. Your client has CHF and has come to you for a massage. The client states that his doctor recommended the massage. You should
    A. perform the massage.
    B. do light Swedish.
    C. focus on strokes towards the heart to help with blood flow.
    D. not perform the massage.

15. Physical or emotional harm sustained by the client due to lack of knowledge or insensitivity on the therapist's behalf is called
    A. client neglect.
    B. client abuse.
    C. client carelessness.
    D. harassment.

16. Within a year after establishment, NCBTMB was accredited by the
    A. Occupational Safety and Health Administration (OSHA).
    B. National Organization for Competency Assurance (NOCA).
    C. American Massage Therapy Association (AMTA).
    D. Associated Bodywork and Massage Professionals (ABMP).

17. Which of the following is an example of unethical behavior
    A. chewing gum during the massage.
    B. accepting phone calls during a massage session.
    C. discussing a client with another client.
    D. running late for your appointment, again.

18. A client trips over the rug in your waiting room and sprains her wrist. Which type of your insurance would cover the fall?
    A. general liability
    B. medial liability
    C. disability
    D. None, the client needs to file with her own insurance company.

19. Sometimes as you massage, you may notice the client's body repeatedly becoming tense. You may need to
    A. stop the massage.
    B. ask the client directly for feedback.
    C. perform light effleurage for a few strokes.
    D. not worry about it since the client has not said anything.

20. In general, during the massage session
    A. talk only when answering the client's questions or when addressing the client's needs.
    B. tell the client that the quieter he or she is, the more he or she will enjoy the massage.
    C. use this as a time to catch up with your client.
    D. All of the above are correct.

21. Telling the client that you are going to leave the room so she may disrobe in private and that you will knock before you reenter the room
    A. helps to signal the time for the client to get on the massage table.

B. helps her to hurry so that she receives a good full hour massage.

C. alleviates any apprehension she may have about your unannounced reentry to the room.

D. signals the beginning of the massage.

22. Which of the following is NOT recommended as a way to safeguard your client's jewelry and valuables during a massage?
   A. suggest not wearing any jewelry to the massage
   B. place them in your pants pocket for safe keeping
   C. provide a basket or bowl in the room for the client to put them in
   D. provide a locker or locked box to store the items during the massage

23. Before beginning the massage, the therapist may choose to ground and center him/herself by using which of the following techniques?
   A. breathing and body movements
   B. burning incense
   C. spraying aromatherapy in the room
   D. All of the above are correct.

24. As your client is leaving, it is a good idea to
   A. get feedback about the massage session.
   B. ask her if she would prefer to rebook now or call for her next appointment.
   C. send her home with stretches to work on.
   D. All of the above are correct.

25. When you arrive at your massage therapy office, to which of the following should you attend?
   A. check your answering machine, taking care of any calls
   B. look over your schedule and review any client intake forms from your files
   C. clean all massage equipment and prepare the room
   D. All of the above are correct.

26. When you greet your client at the door, you should
   A. introduce yourself if this is the client's first time meeting you.
   B. compliment her on her hair and attire.

C. greet her using her name.
D. Both A and C are correct.

27. As a sole proprietor, the Schedule SE form is used for
   A. quarterly estimated taxes.
   B. year-end tax return.
   C. only when showing a profit.
   D. nothing; is not used by sole proprietors.

28. The 1099 form is a statement used to notify the IRS of
   A. estimated quarterly taxes.
   B. employee wages.
   C. social security deductions.
   D. independent contractor wages.

29. A code of ethics can be defined as
   A. governing laws.
   B. business practices.
   C. moral principles.
   D. standard of care.

30. According to the IRS, which item is taxable?
   A. gifts
   B. bartered services
   C. supplies
   D. charitable contributions

31. Professional liability insurance provides protection against possible
   A. harassment.
   B. job discrimination.
   C. injuries sustained by the client.
   D. injuries sustained by the therapist.

32. Who must submit a Schedule C tax statement to the IRS?
   A. Partnership corporations
   B. Salaried employees
   C. S-corporations
   D. Sole proprietor businesses

33. The overall income generated by a business minus expenses is called
   A. gross income.
   B. net income.
   C. overhead.
   D. fiscal finances.

34. According to the NCBTMB Code of Ethics, draping is for
    A. ensuring safety, comfort, and privacy.
    B. providing warmth.
    C. more for the client than it is for the therapist.
    D. preventing sexual and inappropriate incidences.

35. The easiest and least expensive way to incorporate is
    A. partnership.
    B. sole proprietorship.
    C. S-corporation.
    D. corporation.

36. The best form of marketing that is the least expensive is
    A. business cards.
    B. flyers on cars in the parking lot.
    C. word-of-mouth.
    D. small ad in the newspaper.

37. In order to utilize your advertising best, you should
    A. offer qualifiers such as deadlines and expiration dates in your ads.
    B. discuss why your competitor is not qualified.
    C. advertise everywhere possible to get the maximum clients.
    D. put most of your budget into advertising.

38. Which of the following would NOT count as a mileage tax deduction?
    A. mileage from your home to your clinic location
    B. mileage from the office supply store to pick up your business cards to your first client of the day
    C. mileage from your first client back to your outside-of-the-home massage clinic/office
    D. mileage from the post office to drop off business mailings to a meeting with a chiropractor about your massage practice

39. Which of the following is important in preventing burn-out?
    A. exercise
    B. attending continuing education

C. scheduling time off regularly
D. all are important

40. A _____ is someone who renders aid or performs a service without direct monetary gain. It is done of his or her own free will, usually in the sense of charity.
    A. therapist
    B. volunteer
    C. client
    D. contractor

41. Some of the positive aspects of insurance reimbursements are
    A. fee payments set by the insurance company that are competitive with the going rates.
    B. time delay in receipt of reimbursement.
    C. greater professional respect by networking with physicians and attorneys.
    D. Both A and C are correct.

42. Important business resources include a variety of business and civic organizations such as the
    A. public library.
    B. Service Core of Retired Executives.
    C. Small Business Association.
    D. All of the above are correct.

43. A written agreement between two or more parties that outlines expectations, duties, and responsibilities and is enforceable by law is a/an
    A. curriculum vitae.
    B. contract.
    C. proposal.
    D. opportunity.

44. The guidelines for writing a mission statement
    A. are short in length and in accord with your values.
    B. should focus on the needs of other people.
    C. are approved by someone you respect.
    D. Both A and B are correct.

45. What is a mission statement?
    A. a statement of purpose
    B. a bill of therapists' rights
    C. the title of your business
    D. your code of ethics

46. Managing incoming calls and telephone communications is called
    A. secretarial work.
    B. telephone etiquette.
    C. electronic secretary.
    D. office etiquette.

47. One-time start-up costs do NOT include which of the following?
    A. salaries
    B. equipment and machinery
    C. room furnishings
    D. utility deposits

48. This type of insurance is also referred to as malpractice insurance and covers liability costs rising from our professional activities
    A. professional liability.
    B. general liability.
    C. business personal property.
    D. disability insurance.

49. Which of the following types of insurance provides you with income in the event that you cannot work due to extended illness or injury?
    A. professional liability
    B. general liability
    C. business personal property
    D. disability insurance

50. Also referred to as premise liability, this type of insurance takes care of liability costs that are the result of trips and falls within your clinic/office or property damage
    A. professional liability.
    B. general liability.
    C. business personal property.
    D. disability insurance.

51. Having integrity is
    A. the condition of being whole and undivided.
    B. dealing honestly with yourself and with others.
    C. subscribing to a value system and adhering to it.
    D. All of the above are correct.

52. Image is referred to as a/an
    A. mental and emotional portrayal of you in the public eye.
    B. instantaneous impression or picture of you when your name is brought up.
    C. illustration or photograph of yourself.
    D. Both A and B are correct.

53. Which of the following tax forms is filed by the self-employed contractor?
    A. W-2
    B. 1040ES
    C. 1099 form
    D. self-employed do not have to file if paid in cash

54. Things to remember in order to lessen your liability as a massage therapist include all of the following except
    A. when in doubt, refer it out.
    B. it's all connected.
    C. do no harm.
    D. if it is not written in the SOAPs, you cannot be held responsible.

55. The athletic trainer tells you not to work on one of his athletes. The athlete comes to you anyway. What should you do?
    A. work on the athlete since it's up to him/her anyway
    B. talk to the coach and if it's OK with him/her, do the massage
    C. doesn't matter since massage won't hurt the athlete
    D. follow the athletic trainer's directions

56. When a therapist takes a history and performs a physical assessment to identify benefits of treatment, this is called a
    A. medical clearance.
    B. informed consent.
    C. needs assessment.
    D. SOAP charting.

57. Your client states that he has a low backache after working out in his yard. This would go into what section of the SOAP chart?
    A. S
    B. O
    C. A
    D. P

58. The client has a medical condition. Telling the client that he needs to see his doctor would go into what section of the SOAP chart?
    A. S
    B. O
    C. A
    D. P

59. Your client has come to you with shin pain. He or she points to a particular spot. You state, "You have a stress fracture." You, as the therapist, have just
    A. assisted your client in determining the need for a doctor.
    B. stepped outside of your scope of work.
    C. found an injury that can be treated with massage.
    D. improved your therapist/client relationship and trust.

60. Your neighbor has received several massages from you in order to help her with a diagnosed medical condition (she has received clearance to get massages from her physician). A mutual friend asks about her, and you tell her about the diagnosis. You have
    A. violated confidentiality.
    B. not violated confidentiality because you are all friends.
    C. violated your client's informed consent.
    D. stepped outside of your scope of practice.

61. Why is continuing education important for professional ethics?
    A. it helps to promote business
    B. it helps set a higher standard and maintains/improves knowledge
    C. it is necessary in order to be a member of massage organizations
    D. it really isn't important to professional ethics

62. When is it inappropriate to disclose confidential client information?
    A. when required by court order
    B. when requested by the IRS
    C. when the spouse of the client requests
    D. when the client requests

63. Independent contractors submit which year-end wage and tax statement to IRS?
    A. 1099 form
    B. 1040ES
    C. W-2 form
    D. None, because independent contractors do not need to submit year-end forms.

64. Which type of physician is able to diagnose mental disorders?
    A. psychiatrist
    B. psychologist
    C. physiologist
    D. phlebotomist

65. What should you do if a new client refuses to complete the intake form?
    A. refuse the massage
    B. proceed with the massage
    C. ask questions to the client to get as much information as possible
    D. reschedule the massage

66. The S in SOAP stands for
    A. symptoms.
    B. signs.
    C. subjective.
    D. syndrome.

67. Professional ethics can be defined as
    A. following legal and business standards.
    B. promotion of public welfare, client's welfare, and the professional reputation.
    C. marketing techniques.
    D. providing excellent service.

68. Failure to do what you should do, or failure to not do what you should not do is called
    A. ignorance.
    B. low liability risk.
    C. harassment.
    D. negligence.

69. When massaging a client with a potentially fatal disease, the main concern is
    A. keeping the massage within the length that the client can handle.
    B. the emotional state of the client.
    C. advice of the attending physician.
    D. type of strokes necessary for the client.

70. Even though massage therapists are not counselors, a therapist can
    A. advise clients on personal matters.
    B. tell the client how he or she should handle his or her emotions.
    C. find a test on the Internet for the client to take to determine if he or she is depressed.
    D. support the client emotionally and refer out when needed.

71. When your client is in a wheelchair, you should
    A. sit down in a chair so you can speak to him at eye level.
    B. inquire about his limitations.
    C. be prepared to massage him while he is in his wheelchair if necessary.
    D. All of the above are correct.

72. When a client has a healing crisis from a foot reflexology session, this would be noted where in the SOAP notes?
    A. S
    B. O
    C. A
    D. P

Answers and Explanations

Professional Standards, Ethics, and Business and Legal Practices
NCETM (6%)   NCETMB (6%)

1. **A** This is a review of NCBTMB Code of Ethics.

2. **D** All of the above are necessary.

3. **D** Sixty to seventy degrees would be too cold for the client; seventy to eighty degrees and seventy-eight to eighty-five degrees would be too warm for client and therapist. Sixty-eight to seventy-five degrees is a good compromise for both therapist and client.

4. **D** Eclampsia can lead to toxemia and can be life-threatening to both mother and child.

5. **A** This is a review of NCBTMB Code of Ethics.

6. **D** This is a review of NCBTMB requirements.

7. **C** Confidentiality means that information discussed either in writing or verbally will not be discussed by the therapist without expressed written consent of the client.

8. **D** All of these help determine the pricing you choose for your services.

9. **C** Revenue is the taxable item that taxes must be paid.

10. **A** The others involve governmental oversight.

11. **C** Social security numbers are not necessary in an incident report.

12. **B** In order to be viewed by the IRS as a separate entity, you must BE a separate entity. Therefore, you must incorporate yourself, get your own business license, and set up a separate business account.

13. **A** "D" would get you in some hot water! "A" is required by IRS tax laws.

14. **D** Just because a client says his doctor recommended the massage doesn't mean it really happened. Any lawyer will tell you, "If it's not in writing, it didn't happen." Defer the massage until you can get something in writing from the doctor handling the heart treatment that says massage is OK.

15. **A** Negligence is failure to do what is appropriate or to act properly.

16. **B** This is a little history!

17. **C** The others are examples of unprofessional behavior but not unethical behavior.

18. **A** General liability covers trips and falls; business personal property covers property items; disability insurance covers the therapist if he or she is injured and cannot work by providing some sort of income. Professional liability covers the therapist if the client claims the therapist injured him or her during the massage.

19. **B** Sometimes clients are apprehensive about saying anything about the pressure, so it is best to ask if the pressure is OK and modify if necessary.

20. **A** How much talking is done during the session is up to the client, not the therapist. Some clients benefit from talking, but that is up to the client.

21. **C** This is especially true for the new, beginner client.

22. **B** These items can fall out of your pocket or be forgotten, and you could take them home by accident.

23. **A** The question is asking how to ground the therapist, not the client. The other methods might be useful for the client . . . or not.

24. **D** By doing all of these, you are demonstrating to your client the importance of self-care while helping your business to grow by scheduling another appointment to fit her needs. It also helps to ensure the client will come back by scheduling right after the session to ensure she is receiving the treatment she needs.

25. **D** This ensures prompt phone call returns while making sure you are aware of your first client and are prepared for him or her.

26. **D** Meet and greet are the first steps to establishing rapport.

27. **B** As a sole proprietor you pay self-employment taxes and quarterly/annual income. Because you may have paid too much or too little tax due to annual income fluctuations, you may owe more or be due a refund. The schedule SE also allows you to file deductions. Remember, sole proprietors are using their own social security number as their business in most cases. Sole proprietors file a Schedule C with their 1040 forms.

28. **D** Estimated quarterly tax is the 1040 form; the W-4 form is used to report employee wages.

29. **C** Ethics is defined as principles of right and good conduct. Therefore, a code of ethics is what is deemed right and good conduct for massage therapists and bodyworkers by a governing or certification organization such as NCBTMB.

30. **B** The other three choices have a minimum tax deduction already given.

31. **C** Injuries sustained by the therapist would be covered under disability insurance in the event the therapist is unable to work.

32. **A** Schedule C tax form (also known as a 1040 form) is used by sole proprietors and contractors to report income.

33. **B** Gross income is all revenue generated. Overhead is expenses only, but subtract overhead from gross and you have net income.

34. **A** This is a review of the NCBTMB Code of Ethics.

35. **B** The others are more expensive.

36. **C** Word-of-mouth does not cost a thing.

37. **A** Never put down the competition—talk yourself up instead. Getting the maximum number of clients may not be feasible if you are a small business. Also, the demographics may not be conducive to your location if you advertise in a broad area. Most of your budget should be for salary, not marketing.

38. **A** According to the IRS, everyone has to get from home to work and vice versa, so this mileage is not tax deductible.

39. **D** Enough said here!

40. **B** No payment means you are volunteering your time.

41. **D** Unfortunately with insurance reimbursements, you do not receive your payment until a later time, sometimes weeks or months. This is a negative aspect.

42. **D** The library has local listings of businesses and educational books about business; "B" and "C" will help provide contacts and connections.

43. **B** Key words are "written agreement" and "enforceable by law."

44. **D** Approval by someone you respect is helpful but not a basic guideline in the writing of it.

45. **A** A mission statement is explaining to yourself as well as others why you are doing what you're doing.

46. **B** Good telephone etiquette is a must.

47. **A** One-time start-up costs are just what they say . . . one-time costs. Salaries are an ongoing expense.

48. **A** General liability covers trips and falls; business personal property covers property items; disability insurance covers the therapist if he or she is injured and cannot work by providing some sort of income. Professional liability covers the therapist if he or she injures someone while acting as a massage therapist.

49. **D** General liability covers trips and falls; business personal property covers property items; disability insurance covers the therapist if he or she is injured and cannot work by providing some sort of income. Professional liability covers the therapist if he or she injures someone while acting as a massage therapist.

50. **B** General liability covers trips and falls; business personal property covers property items; disability insurance covers the therapist if he or she is injured and cannot work by providing some sort of income. Professional liability covers the therapist if he or she injures someone while acting as a massage therapist.

51. **D** Integrity is what you would do if no one saw you and no one would find out. All of these answer choices qualify.

52. **D** Image is not a picture but a mental image.

53. **B** The 1099 is for payroll tax. "D" is incorrect because any income must be reported or it is a violation. A W-2 is a form to report income from pensions and retirements (IRAs).

54. **D** Remember, whether you write it down or not, you must still follow your scope of work and your national and state standards.

55. **D** The athletic trainer is a licensed health-care worker. It is the athletic trainer who has priority in the say of an athlete's rehabilitation and treatment; otherwise, you may be placing yourself in a liability situation.

56. **C** Medical clearance is only given by a medical doctor. Informed consent is what the client gives the therapist saying he or she knows the risk and benefits of massage and it is still OK for the therapist to perform one. SOAP charting is the therapist's notes of what was done/said before, during, and after the massage.

57. **A** The **S** is subjective and is what the client states. The **O** is objective and is factual information. The **A** is the action done on the client, and the **P** is the plan—what the recommendations are by the therapist to the client.

58. **D** This is basic SOAP charting. The client's statements go under the **S** for subjective.

59. **B** Therapists cannot diagnose injuries or diseases.

60. **A** You knew of the condition because of a medical clearance provided by her doctor to receive massage. If you were not a massage therapist, you would not have received the clearance or the information about your friend.

61. **B** CECs are not needed to join an association or organization, only if you want to become certified/licensed. CECs are important for promoting business, but the questions asks from an ethical standpoint, so "B" is the better choice.

62. **C** Unless told by legal terms or government terms, all information should be kept confidential unless the client requests it in writing to be given to someone else.

63. **A** This is a review of business forms. Independent contractors submit quarterly and final year-end forms.

64. **A** Psychiatrists are licensed medical professionals who are able to diagnose.

65. **C** As long as you get the information, whether in writing or verbally, you can make a decision on whether the client is medically able to receive a massage. A statement should be noted in the SOAP notes that the client declined to fill out the form but that information was received verbally. Hopefully, the client will complete the form at a later time. In the meantime, the client should at least initial the information the therapist wrote for liability purposes.

66. **C** SOAP is **S**ubjective, **O**bjective, **A**ction, **P**lan.

67. **B** Ethics has to do with appropriate conduct of what is right versus what is wrong.

68. **D** Negligence is failure to do what is appropriate or to act properly.

69. **C** The physician is a vital source of information concerning treatment, medication changes and effects, and timing of the massage in relation to treatments (such as chemotherapy). Communication with the physician is vital.

70. **D** We cannot counsel outside of our scope of practice or diagnose.

71. **D** This shows courtesy to the wheelchair-bound client.

72. **A** This would be a "client states . . ." which is subjective.

Eastern Modalities (only on the NCETMB Exam)

chapter 7

Strategies to Success

Study Skills

Practice repetition! Practice repetition!

One of the most common ways to remember something is to repeat it often. If you have trouble remembering certain material, use any or all of these strategies: (1) Review your notes on the subject; try reading them aloud to yourself. (2) Create flash cards. Carry them with you and test yourself often. (3) Write out summary sheets of the most important terms and concepts you want to remember. The very acts of reading silently, reciting, and writing something over and over again will help you remember when it's time for the exam.

Eastern Terminology

Eastern health theory and the unity of its body-mind-spirit connection is based on the energy of chi.

Ayurveda is a wholistic system of medicine from India. It has a strong connection between the mind and the body. It is understood that energetic forces influence nature and human beings. The person is unique and made up of 5 elements—air, fire, water, earth, and ether.

Chi: Chi (qi) means "life force" or energy that flows through the body. It is the vital force of life.

Hara: In Japanese therapies, the Hara is the belly. This is the center of gravity and the energetic center. In China, three energy centers exist. These are called dantien.

Qi Gong is a practice of harnessing and directing Qi (which is Life Energy) from the Universe and from one's inner self.

Shiatsu was developed in Japan based on the principles of Chinese medicine to restore the body's flow of energy. Shiatsu means "finger pressure."

Tao: Tao means "way" and supports the balanced function of all the senses and teaches a lifestyle of moderation. Tao is the path or way to sustain chi energy.

Tui Na is a Chinese form of bodywork that uses rhythmic compressions along energy channels as well as a variety of techniques that manipulate and lubricate joints. Tui Na directly affects flow of energy by holding and compressing the body at accupressure points.

The Five Element Theory

In Chinese philosophy, the natural world can be classified by the five elements. These are also called the five phases, and there are two cycles that interact.

The generating cycle: In the generating cycle, wood creates fire; fire creates earth; earth creates metal; metal creates water; and water creates wood. See Figure 7-1A.

The control cycle: This cycle provides a balance for the generating cycle. In the control cycle wood controls earth; earth controls water; water controls fire; fire controls metal; metal controls wood. See Figure 7-1B.

In harmony: The generating and control cycles describe the five elements in harmony. When these two cycles are not working properly, one organ system may become depleted, allowing the controlling element to weaken and overwhelm it. If fire is weak, then water may over-control or overact on the fire element. Another pathological interaction occurs when one element becomes so excessive that it rebels against or insults the element that normally controls it. Fire, for example, may insult water by reversing the controlling sequence and vaporizing water. An understanding of this interplay allows the practitioner to tonify or sedate the appropriate organ. See Table 7-1.

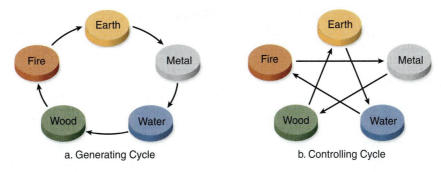

Figure 7-1 The generating and controlling cycles.

TABLE 7-1

At a Glance: Five Element Correspondences

Element	Wood	Fire	Earth	Metal	Water
Season	Spring	Summer	Late summer	Fall	Winter
Process	Birth	Growth	Transformation	Harvest	Storage
Climate	Windy	Hot	Humidity	Dryness	Cold
Color	Green	Red	Yellow/brown	White	Black/blue
Yin organ	Liver	HT/PC*	Spleen	Lungs	Kidneys
Yang organ	Gallbladder	SI/TH*	Stomach	Large intestine	Bladder
Tissue	Muscles	Blood vessels	Flesh	Skin	Bones
Sense	Sight	Speech	Taste	Smell	Hearing
Taste	Sour	Bitter	Sweet	Spicy	Salty
Sound	Shouting	Laughing	Singing	Crying	Groaning
Mental quality	Emotion, sensitivity	Will power, creativity	Compassion, clarity	Intuition	Spontaneity
Negative emotion	Anger	Hate	Anxiety	Grief	Fear
Positive emotion	Patience	Joy	Empathy	Courage	Calmness
Capacity	Planning	Spiritual awareness	Ideas/opinions	Elimination	Ambition

*HT = Heart PC = Pericardium SI = Small Intestine TH = Triple Heater

Yin/yang: Yin and yang are universal characteristics used to describe aspects of the natural world. See Table 7-2. Yin and yang and the five elemental energies form the main roots in the foundation of traditional Chinese medicine. Yang meridians run down the posterior side of the body; yin meridians run up the anterior side of the body.

Meridians: Meridians are channels through which energy flows that are internally associated with organs and externally associated with the surface of the head, trunk, and extremities. See Table 7-3. In these generating and controlling cycles, your internal organs play a dual role in promoting and maintaining your health—generating and regulating energy for each other. Each organ passes energy to the organ it supports, and, when necessary, controls imbalances in the energy of the organ that it regulates. All meridians start or finish in the head, chest, hands, or feet (Figure 7-2). The "solid" organs are involved primarily in collecting, storing, and circulation. These are the yin organs. The corresponding yang organs are "hollow" organs and deal mainly with functions of movement, digestion, and transformation. Another principle to remember is that each of the six pairs of organs is governed by one of the five elemental energies (as noted on Figure 7-1).

TABLE 7-2

At a Glance: Yin/Yang Aspects

Yin	Yang
Feminine	Masculine
Dark	Light
Cold	Hot
Moist	Dry
Earth	Heaven
Soft tissue	Hard tissue
Deficiency	Excess
Dull pain	Sharp pain
Pale tongue	Red tongue
Water	Fire
Team/community	Competitive
Anterior	Posterior

Figure 7-2 The meridians.

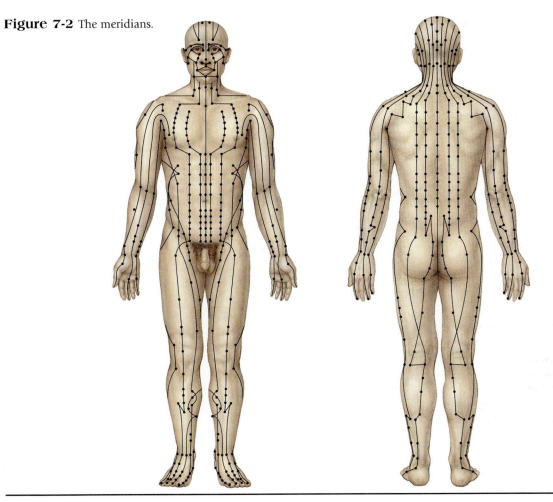

TABLE 7-3

At a Glance: Meridians

Meridian	Location	Yin or Yang
1. Lung	Starts on chest in front of shoulder, finishes in thumb	Yin
2. Large Intestine	Starts in index finger, finishes at side of nostril	Yang
3. Stomach	Starts under eye, finishes in second toe	Yang
4. Spleen	Starts in big toe, finishes at side of chest	Yin
5. Heart	Starts under armpit, finishes in little finger	Yin
6. Small Intestine	Starts in little finger, finishes in front of ear	Yang
7. Urinary Bladder	Starts at inside corner of eye, finishes in little toe	Yang
8. Kidney	Starts on sole of foot, finishes at top of chest	Yin
9. Heart Constrictor	Starts beside nipple, finishes in middle finger	Yin
10. Triple Heater	Starts in fourth finger, finishes by outside corner of eyebrow	Yang
11. Gall Bladder	Starts at outside corner of eye, finishes in fourth toe	Yang
12. Liver	Starts in big toe, finishes on front of chest or below nipple.	Yin
Governing vessel (unpaired)	Tip of tailbone, up midline of back and over the heart to upper lip	Yang
Conception vessel (unpaired)	Perineum and up front of midline to bottom lip and chin	Yin

Meridians also have a time of day that they are most active (Table 7-4). For every two hours throughout the day, one organ-channel is at its peak while the organ opposite that hour (e.g., bladder/lungs) is at its low.

TABLE 7-4

At A Glance: The Twelve Meridians and Corresponding Elements

Meridians	Paired Organ	Color	Peak Hours	Functions and Influences	Psycho-emotional Aspects
Stomach (earth/yang)	Spleen	Deep yellow	7 A.M.–9 A.M.	Digestion, absorption of postnatal energy, mental state	Agitate the mind, mania, hypomania, confusion, severe anxiety, hyperactivity
Spleen (earth/yin)	Stomach	Orange yellow	9 A.M.–11 A.M.	Cleanses and "modifies" blood; thoughts, intention, analytical thinking, trust, honesty, openness, acceptance	Worry, excessive thinking, pensiveness, obsessiveness, remorse, regret, obsessions, and self-doubt
Heart (fire/yin)	Small intestine	Red with slight blue tint	11 A.M.–1 P.M.	Pulse/circulation, house of the spirit; dominates sleep, love, joy, forgiveness, courtesy	Inability to fall asleep, disturbed sleep, excessive dreaming; guilt, hate, shock, nervousness, excitement, longing, craving
Small intestines (fire/yang)	Heart	Pink	1 P.M.–3 P.M.	Absorbs nutrients, digestion and elimination; mental clarity, judgment, powers of discernment	Inability to distinguish relevant issues with clarity before making a decision
Bladder (water/yang)	Kidneys	Deep blue	3 P.M.–5 P.M.	Stores and eliminates urine	Habitual fear, lack of decision making, diminished moral character. When chronic, jealousy, suspicion, holding long-standing grudges
Kidney (water/yin)	Bladder	Light flame blue	5 P.M.–7 P.M.	Controls sexual and reproductive functions, filters the blood; courage and willpower, drive and strength	Fear and paranoia, loneliness, insecurity
Pericardium (fire/yin)	Triple burner	Purple red	7 P.M.–9 P.M.	Protects the heart; creates feelings of joy and/or pleasure	Radical fluctuations in energy caused by every emotional up and down of the day
Triple burner (fire/yang)	Pericardium	Orange red	9 P.M.–11 P.M.	Regulates transformation and transportation of bodily fluids; lifts depression, consciousness, kindheartedness	Disharmony, depression, sadness
Gallbladder (wood/yang)	Liver	Yellow green	11 P.M.–1 A.M.	Stores and excretes bile, one of the extraordinary organs; decisions and judgment, courage and initiative	Wake up suddenly, timid, indecisive, easily discouraged by slight adversity

TABLE 7-4 CONTINUED

Meridians	Paired Organ	Color	Peak Hours	Functions and Influences	Psycho-emotional Aspects
Liver (wood/yin)	Gallbladder	Deep green	1 A.M.– 3 A.M.	Stores the blood, governs the free flow of qi; kindness, compassion, generosity, creativity	Frustration, jealousy, rage, depression, anger, irritability
Lung (metal/yin)	Large intestine	Pure white	3 A.M.– 5 A.M.	Accepts pure fluids from spleen, which are then mixed with air and circulated through the meridians; self-protection, self-preservation, righteousness, dignity, integrity, high self-esteem	Disappointment, sadness, grief, despair, anxiety, shame, and sorrow
Large intestines (metal/ yang)	Lungs	Off white	5 A.M.– 7 A.M.	Absorption of fluids, elimination of solid waste	Physical weakness, emotional introversion, depression, irritability, discouragement, distress, apathy

Chakras: Chakras store and activate our emotions and emotional responses. If a chakra is in balance, we are able to deal effectively with whatever comes our way. If a chakra is blocked or out of balance, we are not able to handle things as well because our perspective is restricted by the condition of the chakra. Each of the seven chakras plays a vital role in our physical body and in our normal subjective consciousness. The chakras are the means by which the functions are carried out. There is generally overlapping and sharing of functions with chakras. See Table 7-5 for physiological and psychological components of chakras.

TABLE 7-5

At a Glance: Chakras of Ayurveda

Chakra	Organ	Element	Color	Emotion
1. Base or root	Spine	Earth	Red	Survival, physical relationships, concepts, patterns, fight or flight
2. Spleen	Gonads	Water	Orange	Relationships, expression of emotions, pleasure, movement, sensation
3. Solar plexus	Muscles, adrenal glands, liver, spleen, gallbladder, lumbar vertebrae, pancreas	Fire	Yellow	Metabolic energy through the body, personal empowerment
4. Heart	Heart thymus gland, endocrine, circulatory systems	Air	Green (sometimes pink)	Ability to express love and unconditional love
5. Throat	Thyroid, parathyroid, neck	Ether	Blue	Communication, higher creativity
6. Third eye	Eyes, ears, nose, pineal gland, pituitary gland	Light	Indigo	Light, color, seeing, greatest teacher of fear and love
7. Crown center	Pituitary gland	Fohat	Violet	Mind and brain

Tsubos: Meridians themselves do not begin or end on the outside of the body but originate deep within the organs and vital energetic centers (chakras) of the body. So, by modifying the energy point just beneath the surface of the skin, we are modifying the energy deep within the body. The acupuncture point for this is called a *tsubo*. Tsubos can be connected to several meridians and interact with energy inside as well as outside the body. It can also be said that chakras are like giant tsubo points. Tsubos are reactive points in Japanese modalities, what some would think of as trigger points in Western modalities.

Acupoints: Acupoints are points on the body that influence or are influenced by body energy. They are named according to the meridian they follow.

Ashi points: Ashi points are reactive points in Chinese modalities.

Eastern Modality Assessments

Now let's pull some of this together for assessment techniques. Clients are assessed by looking, listening/smelling, answering questions, and palpating.

- *Look* at the client to observe overall demeanor, mobility, posture, facial expressions, color, shape, fingernails, and especially the tongue.
- *Listen* to the client to hear what he or she is saying but also what he or she is not saying. Pay attention to the sound of the voice or the odor of the breath, and relate it back to the five elements.
- *Ask* questions about appetite, eating habits, sleep patterns, and energy level highs and lows. Asking the client instead of only filling out an intake form allows the therapist to "look and listen" to the client.
- *Palpate* in order to feel the quality of energy, temperature, moisture levels, tonicity, and other features that are noteworthy.

Yin and yang should be in balance, but when one is overactive, the correspondences on Table 7-4 take over. This throws the body out of homeostasis. The goal of many Eastern modality sessions is to unblock the congestion so the flow of chi (qi) can be achieved and balance can be resumed.

Pathologies in Eastern Medicine

While two people can have the same problems, they might be treated differently depending on the manifestation of the disorder. See Table 7-6 for manifestations of disease and the corresponding meridian. In no way is this meant to be for diagosis.

TABLE 7-6

At a Glance: Pathologies and Meridians

Median	Manifestation
Lung Meridian	Hemoptysis, cough, asthma, congested and sore throat, a sensation of fullness in the chest. Pain in the supraclavicular fossa, shoulder, back, and anterior border of the medial aspect of the arm, heat in the wrist and/or palms, shortness of breath, enuresis, and frequency of urination
Large Intestine Meridian	Epistaxis, watery nasal discharge, toothache, congested and sore throat, and pain in the neck, anterior part of the shoulder, and anterior border of the lateral aspect of the upper limb, abdominal pain, diarrhea and dysentery, toothache and/or coldness in the teeth, deafness, a feeling of compression in the chest and/or diaphragm
Stomach Meridian	Abdominal distension, edema, epigastric pain, vomiting, hunger, epistaxis, deviation of the mouth, congested and sore throat, pain in the chest, abdomen, and lateral aspect of the lower limbs, fever and mania, emotional disorder such as depression or manic behavior, muscular atrophy, weakness in the lower limb or atrophy, congested and sore throat, sudden hoarseness
Spleen Meridian	Belching, vomiting, epigastric pain, abdominal distension, loose stools, jaundice, heaviness of the body, lassitude, stiffness and pain in the root of the tongue, swelling and coldness in the medial aspect of the thigh, abdominal spasm, cholera with vomiting and/or diarrhea
Heart Meridian	Cardiac pain, palpitations, hypochondriac pain, insomnia, night sweating, dryness of the throat, thirst, pain in the medial aspect of the upper arm, heat sensation in the palms, fullness in the chest and/or diaphragms, aphasia
Small Intestine Meridian	Deafness, yellow sclera, sore throat, swelling of the cheeks, distension and pain in the lower abdomen, pain in the posterior border of the lateral aspect of the shoulder and arm, weakness of the joints, muscular atrophy, motor impairment of the elbow, warts on the skin
Bladder Meridian	Retention of urine, enuresis, manic and depressive mental disorders, malaria, pain in the eyes, lacrimation when exposed to wind, nape of the neck, back, lower back, buttocks, and posterior aspect of the lower limbs, nasal congestion, watery nasal discharge, headache, pain in the back along the channel, and epistaxis
Kidney Meridian	Frequent urination, nocturnal emission, impotence, irregular menstruation, asthmatic breathing, hemoptysis, dryness of the tongue, congested and sore throat, edema, pain in the lumbar region, pain in the posteromedial aspect of the thigh, weakness in the lower limbs, heat sensation in the soles, retention of urine, low back pain, mental restlessness, chest oppression
Pericardium Meridian	Cardiac pain, palpitations, mental restlessness, stuffiness in the chest, flushed face, swelling in the axilla, depressive and manic mental disorders, spasm of the upper limbs and heat sensation in the palms, cardiac pain, mental restlessness
Triple Burner Meridian	Abdominal distension, edema, enuresis, dysuria, deafness, tinnitus, swelling of the cheeks, congested and sore throat, pain in the retro auricular region, shoulder, and lateral aspect of the chest, hypochondrium, thigh and lower limbs, either spastic or flaccid cubital joint
Liver Meridian	Low back pain, fullness in the chest, pain in the lower abdomen, hernia, vertical headache, dryness of the throat, hiccups, enuresis, dysuria, mental disturbance, itching in the pubic region, swelling of the testicles, hernia
Gallbladder Meridian	Headache, pain in the jaw, blurring of vision, bitter taste in the mouth, swelling and pain in the supraclavicular fossa, pain in the axilla, pain along the lateral aspect of the chest, hypochondrium, thigh and lower limbs, coldness in the foot, paralysis in the lower limbs, inability to stand erect

Strategies to Success

Test-Taking Strategy

Come prepared!

Always bring all the supplies you need to the exam. Bring a few number two pencils and a working eraser. Do not depend on someone else to give these supplies to you. Make sure you have two forms of identification (ID). Primary ID: driver's license or other government-issued photo ID. Secondary ID: credit/debit/ATM/check card or military photo ID. Social security cards are not acceptable. Take few deep breaths—good luck!

*Some questions are not directly addressed in this chapter, but are meant to act as a general review of subjects studied in various school curriculums.

Questions

Eastern Modalities (NCBTMB Exam Only)

1. When considering the five elements in Eastern medicine, the food flavor that goes with water is
   A. sweet.
   B. bitter.
   C. sour.
   D. salty.

2. When considering the five elements in Eastern medicine, the food flavor that goes with metal is
   A. pungent.
   B. sweet.
   C. sour.
   D. salty.

3. In shiatsu, the color related to wood is
   A. red.
   B. green.
   C. yellow.
   D. black.

4. In shiatsu, the earth meridian relates or corresponds to which organ?
   A. liver
   B. spleen
   C. heart
   D. lungs

5. Which meridian in Eastern medicine runs down the body and ends at the second toe?
   A. large intestines
   B. small intestines
   C. bladder
   D. stomach

6. Yang meridians run
   A. down the posterior side of the body.
   B. up the posterior side of the body.
   C. down the anterior side of the body.
   D. up the anterior side of the body.

7. In shiatsu, the hara is located in the
   A. abdomen.
   B. meridians.
   C. tsubos.
   D. heart.

8. In the five element theory of Eastern medicine, the earth element consists of what yin component?
   A. lung
   B. spleen
   C. bladder
   D. stomach

9. What are the five elements in Eastern medicine?
   A. wood, fire, earth, metal, water
   B. earth, wind, fire, metal, water
   C. wood, wind, metal, fire, earth
   D. wood, air, metal, fire, wind

10. Yin meridians run
    A. down the anterior side of the body.
    B. up the anterior side of the body.
    C. down the posterior side of the body.
    D. up the posterior side of the body.

11. In Eastern medicine, which meridian is not paired?
    A. the liver
    B. the large intestines
    C. the conception vessel
    D. the triple heater

12. The solar plexus chakra is related to
    A. circulation.
    B. sexual function.
    C. digestion.
    D. lungs and voice.

13. Kyo-jitsu theory is the study of
    A. Zen.
    B. acupuncture/pressure.
    C. hemostatic patterns of Chi.
    D. all Eastern medicine.

14. The basic technique used in reflexology is the
    A. walking technique
    B. tsubo technique.
    C. acupuncture.
    D. None of the above are correct.

15. There are many times during reflexology treatments when a client experiences a headache or an increase of elimination through the skin, bowels, or urinary system. He/she may even experience a flare-up of an illness that never really resolved. All of these symptoms can be classified as a
    A. chronic illness.
    B. malignancy.
    C. too-deep treatment.
    D. healing crisis.

16. The seventh chakra is called the
    A. solar plexus.
    B. crown center.
    C. heart chakra.
    D. throat chakra.

17. When working on a reflex point, it is better to
    A. use steady pressure.
    B. undertreat than overtreat.
    C. use intermittent pressure.
    D. use deep friction.

18. When looking at the five elements of Eastern medicine, the food flavor that goes with earth is
    A. sweet.
    B. sour.
    C. bitter.
    D. pungent.

19. The main role of the heart channel energy is to
    A. interpret and adapt one to his or her emotional environment.
    B. provide nurturing substances necessary for a creative life.
    C. motivate.
    D. affect the feelings of self-worth.

20. When looking at the five element theory in Eastern medicine, the food flavor that goes with fire is
    A. sour.
    B. sweet.
    C. pungent.
    D. bitter.

21. Balancing energy systems and polarity are addressed by
    A. Shiatsu.
    B. Rolfing.
    C. Hellerwork.
    D. Bindegewebmassage.

22. The stomach Zen channel represents
    A. the ability to release.
    B. nurturing, fertility, and groundedness.
    C. impetus and flexibility.
    D. purification.

23. The Eastern expression "overuse the mind and underuse the body" indicates an imbalance of what element?
    A. wood
    B. fire
    C. earth
    D. water

Answers and Explanations

Eastern Modalities (NCBTMB Exam Only)

1. **D** Wood is sour, fire is bitter, earth is sweet, metal is pungent, and water is salt.

2. **A** Wood is sour, fire is bitter, earth is sweet, metal is pungent, and water is salt.

3. **B** Red is fire, black is water, and yellow is earth.

4. **B** The liver is wood, the heart is fire, and the lungs are metal.

5. **D** Large intestine starts in index finger and finishes at the side of the nostril; small intestine starts in little finger and finishes in front of the ear; and urinary bladder starts at the inside corner of the eye and finishes in the little toe.

6. **A** Yang meridians run down the posterior side of the body; yin meridians run up the anterior side of the body.

7. **A** In Chinese medicine the hara is known as the Lower Dantian and is located about an inch below the navel. The hara is the root of vital energy as well as the nervous system and muscular energy. It is the furnace that produces life, and at the same time it is the source of life regulating the physiological and spiritual well-being. It is seen as controlling the metabolism of the blood and the organs and producing the qi that flows along our meridians.

8. **B** The lung is a metal yin; the bladder is a water yang; and the stomach is an earth yang.

9. **A** Wood, fire, earth, metal, and water are the five elements.

10. **B** Yang meridians run down the posterior side of the body; yin meridians run up the anterior side of the body.

11. **C** The liver is paired with the gallbladder; the large intestine is paired with the lungs; and the triple heater is paired with the heart/pericardium.

12. **C** The heart chakra is circulation; the sexual function is the root and belly chakras; and the lung and voice is the throat chakra.

13. **C** Kyo means deficiency, and jitsu means excess.

14. **A** Tsubos are blocked energy in shiatsu. Acupuncture is performed with needles and requires a higher level of training and education.

15. **D** A healing crisis is a reaction that occurs when the body tries to eliminate toxins at a faster rate than they can be properly disposed of. The more toxic a bodily system is, the more severe the detoxification, or healing crisis. It is characterized by a temporary increase in symptoms during the cleansing or detoxification process, which may be mild or severe. You may feel worse and therefore conclude that the treatment is not working. But these reactions are instead signs that the treatment is working and that your body is going through the process of cleansing itself of impurities, toxins, and imbalances.

16. **B** The heart chakra is the fourth, the solar plexus is the third, and the throat chakra is the fifth.

17. **B** Remember that these zones are related to areas of the body and/or organs. Overtreating could cause much discomfort for your client during and after the session.

18. **A** Wood is sour, fire is bitter, earth is sweet, metal is pungent, and water is salt.

19. **A** Nurturing and creativity are the liver; motivation is the kidney; and feelings of self-worth are the spleen.

20. **D** Wood is sour; fire is bitter; earth is sweet; metal is pungent; and water is salt.

21. **A** Bindegewebmassage was developed in the 1940s; this is a type of connective tissue massage that follows the patterns of dermatomes. By use of massage in certain patterns and movements, there is a vascular and visceral reflexive effect on many pathologic conditions.

22. **B** The ability to release is the large intestines (elimination); impetus and flexibility are the kidney (it governs the endocrine system); and purification is the urinary bladder.

23. **C** Earth relates to productivity, fertility, and growth. The earth element relates to the stomach (yang) and the spleen (yin). The stomach begins the process of digestive breakdown, while the spleen transforms and transports the energy from food and drink throughout the body. Pensiveness is the emotion that creates imbalance within this element.

Appendix A

Suggested Outline for the NCETMB Prep Course

8:00–8:30 Introductions, Test taking tips
- Basic agenda for test: number of questions, time frame
- How to register for the test
- What to bring to the test/what not to bring
- How to take a standardized test
- Locate the testing center before the test date if possible
- What to do the night before (rest and relax)
- Arriving early for the test

8:30–10:00 General Knowledge of Body Systems (16%)

Anatomy and Physiology
Levels of Organization
- Review of Major Body Systems
- Energy Terminology

The Integumentary System
- Glands of the Integumentary System

The Skeletal System
- Bone Shapes
- Bone Structure
- Major Bones of the Body

The Muscular System

The Nervous System
- Central Nervous System
- Peripheral Nervous System
- Special Senses

The Endocrine System

The Cardiovascular System
- Major Arterial Roots
- Pathologies of Blood Vessels

The Lymph System

The Urinary System

The Respiratory System

The Gastrointestinal System

The Reproductive System
- The Male Reproductive System
- The Female Reproductive System

10:00–10:15 Break

10:15–12:00 Detailed Knowledge of Anatomy, Physiology, and Kinesiology (26%)

Anatomical Position
- Planes of Motion

Cavities of the Body

Body Movements
- Types of Contractions
- Muscle Movers

Biomechanics and Kinesiology
- Muscles
- Joints
- Dermatomes

Nutrition
- The Six Basic Nutrients

12:00–1:00 Lunch

1:00–2:00 Pathology (16%)

Medical Terminology

The Nine Regions of the Abdomen

Risk Factors for Disease

Microorganisms

Modes of Disease Transmission

Stages of Inflammation

Disorders/Diseases
- Massage and Cancer

Drugs and Herbal Therapy

Effects of Physical and Emotional Abuse and Trauma
- Physical Symptoms of Trauma
- Emotional Symptoms of Trauma
- Cognitive Symptoms of Trauma
- Re-experiencing the Trauma
- Emotional Numbing and Avoidance
- Increased Arousal
- Common Personal and Behavioral Effects of Emotional Trauma
- Common Effects of Emotional Trauma on Interpersonal Relationships

2:00–2:15 Break

2:15–3:00 Therapeutic Massage and Bodywork Assessment (18%)

Assessment Methods

Normal Ranges of Motion

Endangerment Sites
- Anterior Triangle of the Neck
- Posterior Triangle of the Neck
- Axillary
- Antecubital Area of Elbow
- Femoral Triangle
- Low Back (Ribs Nine Through Twelve)
- Oleacronon Process Area
- Popliteal Fossa

Postural Analysis

Understanding Kinesiology

Other Factors that Affect the Body

3:00–4:00 Therapeutic Massage Applications (22%)

Effects of Massage
- Physiological Effects
- Emotional Effects
- Psychological Effects

Methods and Techniques of Massage
  Client Draping
  Stress Management and Relaxation
  Other Holistic Techniques
Massage Techniques and Strokes
  Judging Pressure and Depth
  Stretching Techniques
  Practitioner Body Mechanics
Standard Precautions and Procedures
  Hyperthermia
  Pathological Stages of Heat Illness/Injury
  Hypothermia

4:00–4:15 Break

4:15–5:00 Professional Standards, Ethics, Business and Legal Practices (6%)
  The NCBTMB Code of Ethics

Professional Considerations
  Record Keeping
  Planning Single and Multiple Sessions
  Business Concepts
  Types of Business Entities
  Insurance Needs
  Accounting Terms

5:00–6:00 Eastern Modalities
  Eastern Terminology
  Five Elements
  Meridians
  Chakras
  Eastern Modalities Assessments
  Pathology Evaluation

Appendix B

Suggested Outline for the NCETM Prep Course

8:00–8:30 Introductions, Test taking tips
- Basic agenda for test: number of questions, time frame
- How to register for the test
- What to bring to the test/what not to bring
- How to take a standardized test
- Locate the testing center before the test date if possible
- What to do the night before (rest and relax)
- Arriving early for the test

8:30–10:00 General Knowledge of Body Systems (14%)
- Anatomy and Physiology
  - Levels of Organization
  - Review of Major Body Systems
  - Energy Terminology
- The Integumentary System
  - Glands of the Integumentary System
- The Skeletal System
  - Bone Shapes
  - Bone Structure
  - Major Bones of the Body
- The Muscular System
- The Nervous System
  - Central Nervous System
  - Peripheral Nervous System
  - Special Senses
- The Endocrine System
- The Cardiovascular System
  - Major Arterial Roots
  - Pathologies of Blood Vessels
- The Lymph System
- The Urinary System
- The Respiratory System
- The Gastrointestinal System
- The Reproductive System
  - The Male Reproductive System
  - The Female Reproductive System

10:00–10:15 Break

10:15–12:00 Detailed Knowledge of Anatomy, Physiology, and Kinesiology (26%)
- Anatomical Position
  - Planes of Motion
- Cavities of the Body
- Body Movements
  - Types of Contractions
  - Muscle Movers
- Biomechanics and Kinesiology
  - Muscles
  - Joints
  - Dermatomes
- Nutrition
  - The Six Basic Nutrients

12:00–1:00 Lunch

1:00–2:00 Pathology (14%)
- Medical Terminology
- The Nine Regions of the Abdomen
- Risk Factors for Disease
- Microorganisms
- Modes of Disease Transmission
- Stages of Inflammation
- Disorders/Diseases
  - Massage and Cancer
- Drugs and Herbal Therapy
- Effects of Physical and Emotional Abuse and Trauma
  - Physical Symptoms of Trauma
  - Emotional Symptoms of Trauma
  - Cognitive Symptoms of Trauma
  - Re-experiencing the Trauma
  - Emotional Numbing and Avoidance
  - Increased Arousal
  - Common Personal and Behavioral Effects of Emotional Trauma
  - Common Effects of Emotional Trauma on Interpersonal Relationships

2:00–2:15 Break

2:15–3:00 Therapeutic Massage and Bodywork Assessment (16%)
- Assessment Methods
- Normal Ranges of Motion
- Endangerment Sites
  - Anterior Triangle of the Neck
  - Posterior Triangle of the Neck
  - Axillary
  - Antecubital Area of Elbow
  - Femoral Triangle
  - Low Back (Ribs Nine Through Twelve)
  - Oleacronon Process Area
  - Popliteal Fossa
- Postural Analysis
- Understanding Kinesiology
- Other Factors that Affect the Body

3:00–4:00 Therapeutic Massage Applications (24%)
- Effects of Massage
  - Physiological Effects
  - Emotional Effects
  - Psychological Effects

Methods and Techniques of Massage
Client Draping
Stress Management and Relaxation
Other Holistic Techniques

Massage Techniques and Strokes
Judging Pressure and Depth
Stretching Techniques
Practitioner Body Mechanics

Standard Precautions and Procedures
Hyperthermia
Pathological Stages of Heat Illness/Injury
Hypothermia

4:00–4:15 Break

4:15–5:00 Professional Standards, Ethics, Business and Legal Practices (6%)
The NCBTMB Code of Ethics
Professional Considerations
Record Keeping
Planning Single and Multiple Sessions
Business Concepts
Types of Business Entities
Insurance Needs
Accounting Terms

Index